VACCINATION
Rediscovered

Dedicated to the dairymaids

who held the key

shared it with others

and helped to save millions of lives

and

to the memory

of

Colin and Fred

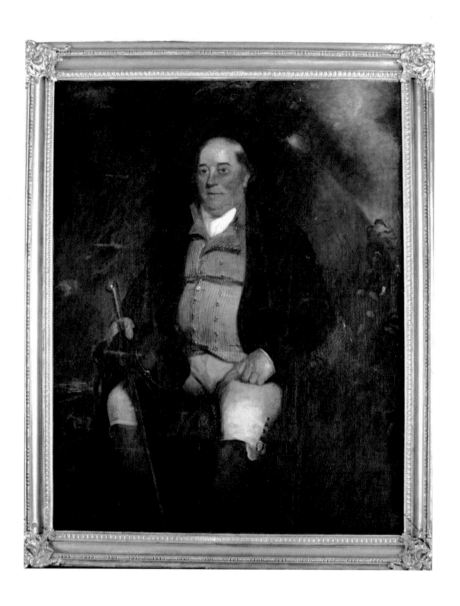

Benjamin Jesty – the first vaccinator

VACCINATION
Rediscovered

New Light in the Dawn
Of Man's Quest for Immunity

Patrick J Pead

Time*f*ile Books
a Division of
Patrick J Pead
Chichester
West Sussex
pjpead@yahoo.co.uk

First published in Great Britain
by Time*f*ile Books in February 2006
This first revision printed in June 2006

A catalogue record for this book
is available from the British Library

Paperback ISBN 0–9551561–0–6

From 1st January 2007 ISBN 978–0–9551561–0–6

Printed and bound in Great Britain by
RPM Print & Design
Chichester, West Sussex, England

Contents

Illustrations

Front cover: 'L'Origine de la Vaccine' an etching by Depeuille, Paris, c1800. A physician examines a cowpox lesion on a milkmaid's hand, while a farmer passes a lancet to another physician.   Wellcome Library, London.

Frontispiece: Benjamin Jesty – the first vaccinator. This portrait in oils completed by Michael W Sharp, London, in 1805, was thought to be lost. The painting was located in South Africa by the author during 2004. It was acquired by the Wellcome Library for the History of Medicine in June 2006.

Acknowledgements

I would like to express my appreciation to all those who assisted me in the production of this manuscript with information, advice, correspondence and much valued encouragement. Many people opened their doors, real or virtual, and told me their stories. Others provided professional opinions on specific questions, or made archival resources available for me to explore:

Margaret Asquith, The Society of Apothecaries of London, Dr Derrick Baxby, Prof Ian Clarke, Michael Clarke, Prof Barry Coller, Dee Cook, Tina Craig, Prof Paul Davis, Dorchester Reference Library, Dorset History Centre, Dorset Life, the late Fred Dowse, Tony Dutton, Pip Firth, John Foster, Linda Garrat, Dr Steve Green, Dr Gamal El Gurashi, Jacqui Halewood, Nina Hayward, Prof John Heckels, Ian Hill, Ron Hill, David Jesty, Prof Jolyon Jesty, Prof Sam Katz, Bryony Kelly, Shirley Laing, Judy Lindsay, Ordnance Survey, Oxford University Press, the late Bernard Pead, John Pead, Charles Pope, the late Christopher Pope, Sylvia Pope, Charles and Mary Roe, Dr Awad Saeed, Ann Smith, Denise and Brian Stickels, Dr and Mrs Sumner, The Lancet, The British Library, The Royal College of Physicians, The Royal College of Surgeons of England, The Wellcome Library for the History of Medicine, The Witt Library, the late Dave Turner, Milton Wainwright, Marjorie Wallace, the late Mary Spencer-Watson, West Sussex Record Office, Michael Windridge, Yetminster Local History Society. Jean Brooks proof-read my first manuscript and I am indebted to Dr Rosalind Maskell who made extremely valuable suggestions for this revised edition.

I am particularly grateful to Bill and Vera Jesty. Some objectives within this project could not have been successfully achieved without their help. I greatly value our strong and lasting friendship.

My very special thanks goes to my dearest wife, Linda, who has accompanied me on this journey of discovery and supported me every step of the way. Her expertise with digital imaging has been invaluable. She has listened, proof-read and advised on so many occasions. Her patience with my continuing research deserves a medal!

Introduction

'History is not what you thought. It is what you can remember'
(1066 and All That)

Before leaving primary school I had already formed the earnest opinion that the past could not provide me with a future. We attempted to learn what we were taught in history lessons and accepted everything that was written in our textbooks. There seemed nothing more to add. My early teenage years coincided with the post-war love affair with science and the career that it promised. When I entered the world of work I nailed the flag of medical science to my masthead and set sail - it was a revelation. Navigating my chosen course, I soon realised that all the waymarks of progress in that speciality were built upon the foundations of what had gone before. The past now became important to me and it mattered that the records were authentic. Whilst I found this was mostly true of the scholarship that I resourced, it seemed that Hermes, the god of science and medicine, had an occasional tendency to be unjust when apportioning credit for achievement in those disciplines.

This book is about the origins of vaccination, but differs from previous titles in attempting to provide the reader with a more comprehensive scenario viewed from a new aspect. The subject is a typical example of those veiled fragilities of history that lurk in the recesses of received wisdom. Many accounts of bygone events were set down for posterity by those who prevailed over others. Some were scripted by members of their families or friends who had a vested interest. Modern retrospective studies have shown that we are left with much archive material where the designated credit is inaccurate, incomplete or totally fabricated. There are examples of historical figures who have gone unrecorded or whose contributions were overlooked. With time, some questionable acknowledgements have become established as sacred truths but in reality they are nothing more than fables set in stone. Sir Francis Darwin was well aware of such anomalies when he delivered the Galton Lecture in 1914, saying 'in science the credit goes to the man who convinces the world, not the man to whom the idea first occurs'. This is singularly unfortunate, for science and technology demand veracity as a fundamental requirement.

The invention of the steam engine is often attributed solely to James Watt, but his actual contribution was to perfect an existing machine devised by Newcomen and Savery. Edmond Halley was not the first to observe Halley's comet, nor did he give it his name. He is celebrated for realising that the comet had a regular periodicity of 76 years and predicting that it would return in 1758. Sir Francis Beaufort's first scale of wind strength was copied from a *Memoir* written by Alexander Dalrymple five years before. Dalrymple, in turn, had adapted an idea proposed by the civil engineer John Smeaton in 1759. It is commonly supposed that Marconi invented radio but this was really the brainchild of the Croat, Nikoli Tesla. The US Supreme Court dismissed Marconi's claim in 1943 when they overturned his patent because it was proven that he had been predated by Tesla. Francis Crick and James Watson will always be remembered for their discovery of the structure of the DNA molecule in 1953. They could not have done this without using data from Rosalind Franklin's X-ray crystallography experiments. Franklin was a far superior chemist; she had worked out the DNA structure independently and was at the point of publication. Crick and Watson's paper reached the presses first, but it did not contain any experimental proofs of their hypothesis, and they failed to acknowledge the all-important contribution of Franklin.

Innovation is by definition always ahead of its time but frequently precipitates the downfall of its proponents. Former victims included Copernicus and Galileo, who were compelled to defer to an omnipotent institution which refused to accept that the Glory of God might be reflected in scientific elegance as well as artistic expression. Although the twentieth century will be remembered as one that heralded innumerable discoveries, Frank Whittle - the inventor of the jet engine - was summarily dismissed by the Air Ministry when he first presented them with his ideas. There were occasions in the history of medicine when intellect was met with total indifference. Prevention of the debilitating effects of scurvy by a regular intake of citrus fruit was first noticed as early as 1534 by Jacques Cartier. This was confirmed seven years later by Sir James Lancaster who gave his sailors a regular issue of lemon juice. His proof was disregarded by the medical establishment of the day, and thousands of seamen were to die of scurvy until James Lind published his recommendations in 1753. Mankind's battle against malaria could have begun in 1572 when the captain of a merchantman noticed that outbreaks of the disease appeared to be associated with mosquito bites. Doctors were not interested, so the world had to wait for three hundred years before this crucial observation was announced by Ronald Ross. He was awarded a Nobel Prize for his work. Later chapters will show how those who introduced the early forms of immunisation were met with disbelief and deep suspicion.

Wainwright has compiled a fascinating review of the deficiencies in 'standard accounts' of discoveries in microbiology. Innumerable textbooks give credit to Louis Pasteur for linking moulds with the process of fermentation, but this work had already been explored in depth (and published) by Antoine Bechamp years before Pasteur began his experiments. In 1849 the physicians Swayne, Britten and Budd, described comma shaped 'fungoid bodies' in the faeces of cholera patients and also reported finding these organisms in water samples from cholera districts. This predated both Pasteur and the father of epidemiology, John Snow, who is noted for associating the infectious nature of water in spreading the disease. Ignatz Semmelweis is hailed as the first to show that hospital epidemics of puerperal fever could be prevented if medical staff washed their hands before attending women in childbirth. Thirty years before Semmelweis, a surgeon named William Hey had adopted this practice at the General Infirmary at Leeds in 1815. He may have based his ideas on the theories of Charles White and Alexander Gordon, who concluded in the late eighteenth century that childbed fever could be reduced by cleanliness and isolation. The American, Oliver Wendell Holmes published a paper in 1843 agreeing with White and Gordon. He mentioned a doctor washing his hands in chloride of lime during maternity visits. Semmelweis wrote about the same topic three years later, so Holmes's earlier publication did nothing to establish his priority. In 1863 an article by the Manchester Professor of Chemistry, Frederick Crace Calvert, was printed in The Lancet. He described the medical uses of carbolic at the Manchester Royal Infirmary, including its use as an antiseptic application to wounds by a surgeon named Thomas Turner. There were other reports of the disinfecting powers of carbolic by McDougall in 1852 and by the Parisian doctor, Lemaire, in 1865. Joseph Lister did not publish his Lancet paper 'On the use of carbolic acid' until 1867, yet he is regarded as the father of antisepsis. In so many cases, the plenary records of our scientific heritage have become usurped by the 'standard accounts' and accepted as historical facts, sometimes to the detriment of truth.

The origins of vaccination are so clouded in myth, that the archives of this branch of medicine are flawed. We are taught that Dr Edward Jenner was the first to 'discover' vaccination when he transferred cowpox material from the hand of Sarah Nelmes to the arm of James Phipps in 1796, but there is now a growing acceptance amongst medical historians that Jenner's priority is a falsehood. Later chapters will describe how Benjamin Jesty, a yeoman farmer from Yetminster in Dorset, preceded Jenner by performing vaccinations to protect his family against smallpox twenty-two years earlier.

I thought I should use the Introduction to explain how I became interested in the subject matter of this book. I spent most of my career as a medical microbiologist, assisting with the diagnosis of infectious diseases in a hospital laboratory at Portsmouth, England, before moving on to research in molecular microbiology at the University of Southampton. My work has always demanded an understanding of how our lives are affected by the world of microbes, why bacteria and viruses are able to overcome our defences and how they can adapt to changes in their environment. Whilst studying for my qualifications I realised how much we owe to the role of vaccines in protecting ourselves against the invisible aggressors that are always in our midst.

During the early part of my career, my late cousin Bernard gave me three photocopied pages from Jenner's epoch-making paper, *An Inquiry into the Causes and Effects of the Variolae Vaccinae* which he self-published in 1798. The extract contained notes relating to the children that were part of his vaccination experiments. Two of them had the names

William Pead and Mary Pead and were entered as cases 20 and 21 respectively in the *Inquiry*. I visited the Gloucester Records Office and found the original scraps of parchment listing the children's baptisms. They were born out of wedlock to their mother, Mary Pead, who lived at Ham, just south of Jenner's home in Berkeley in Gloucestershire. My brother John, the family genealogist, has yet to prove a direct line to these children in our family tree. I hope this will be possible in time as they were involved in the preliminary attempts to defeat the scourge of smallpox, and I have been fortunate to witness the global eradication of that dreadful disease during my own lifetime. I had the good fortune to be admitted as a member of the Jenner Educational Trust in 1996, and on the 20th June of that year my wife and I attended their celebrations at Berkeley to mark the 200th anniversary of Jenner's vaccination of James Phipps. As we entered the Great Hall of Berkeley Castle for the Bicentenary Dinner I felt I was paying a fitting tribute to the participation of William and Mary Pead in Jenner's great work.

My special interest in Benjamin Jesty began by pure chance. Some thirty years ago I was taking a holiday with my wife in Dorset, a county where I spent the early part of my childhood and one which remains close to my heart. We had planned a circular walk in the Isle of Purbeck using the village of Worth Matravers as our starting point. Returning to the village we sought refreshment from the shelves of the local shop. My eye was drawn to a booklet on sale amongst the tourist information. It was entitled 'The First Vaccinator' and the author's name was Marjorie Wallace MA. I purchased a copy immediately. Skimming through this intriguing biography as we ate our lunch, I found her photograph of Jesty's tombstone that stood in the nearby churchyard. We went to see for ourselves. When I read the inscription I knew that Marjorie had started me on a long journey of investigation. More recently I had the great pleasure to meet Mrs Wallace. We talked about our common interest and I found her to possess an agile and enquiring mind that belied her golden years. She expressed great interest in my further researches on Benjamin Jesty. Here was a man forgotten by history, someone whose contribution to medicine had been treated as an irrelevance by the establishment amid the political manoeuvres that surrounded the parliamentary debate for Jenner's rewards in the early 1800s. I began to study the history more closely. The deeper I probed, the more it seemed that the reality had become distorted, like so many milestones in mankind's achievements. Was the 'discovery' of vaccination really just the work of one historical icon at a single time and place, as the textbooks would have us believe, or the culmination of a series of contributions over many years by a number of individuals - pioneers basing their ideas upon notions originating in folklore and practices derived from the mists of antiquity? I decided to investigate.

In this book I want to attempt to paint a wide canvas by introducing new elements into the composition, then view the complete picture from a radical perspective. Today it is fashionable to examine the historical record more critically than ever before. Past events and legendary reputations are often the themes of television documentaries or articles in the media. There is a trend for getting at the truth of our yesterdays and the lessons that might be learnt for our tomorrows. History does not have a monopoly on misrepresentation. We now live in the age of the spin-doctor and there are occasions when it is difficult to have confidence in what we are told by those in high office these days. My intention in writing this book is not to peddle controversy but to produce a balanced opinion which is based on an exploration of my researches over the last thirty years. The viewpoint of my thesis is derived from scholarship, portrayed with sensibility I hope, not sensation. There is absolutely no doubt that Edward Jenner brought the technique of vaccination to the world but the full story of the origins of vaccination spans a broader horizon. We must revisit the eighteenth century to meet three persons from very different backgrounds who all played their part. It is a tale of aristocrats and commoners, of male chauvinism and suppressed intellect, of breathtaking bravado, unrecognized genius and cautious enterprise. **Vaccination Rediscovered** is a chronicle of the earliest pioneers who provided a framework for the pursuit of today's healthcare research in our attempts to seek immunity to infectious and genetically induced diseases. We are forever in their debt.

Please note that I have decided not to include references within the text, to permit an even flow of my narrative. A full bibliography is listed at the end of this book.

Chapter 1

Jabs, Bugs and Rock n Roll

'Just a little prick.' Medicine wears a smile and a crisp uniform. I'm in the treatment room of my GP's surgery, a brightly lit place of sterile packs, bustling efficiency and the whiff of disinfectant. I look away as the needle goes in, for no good reason because it doesn't really hurt – the steel tube is only a fraction of a millimeter in diameter. My Hepatitis A vaccination is over in seconds. 'Don't forget to have a booster in six months time if you want the protection to last for ten years.' The practice nurse bids me goodbye. I drive off in the knowledge that I can look forward to my trip abroad without fear of infection by one of the viruses that might have had designs on my liver.

The phase 'prevention is better than cure' is particularly appropriate when used in the context of infectious diseases. When microbes infect our bodies, they are already causing damage to our organs and tissues by the time we experience the first symptoms. Antibiotics may be effective in halting bacterial invasions but they are powerless against viruses. Although there are situations where some viral diseases can be controlled with chemotherapeutic drugs, the only reason for giving an antibiotic to a patient suffering a virus attack is to ward off the threat of secondary bacterial infection. Unlike bacteria, viruses need to enter the cells which make up our body parts in order to reproduce themselves. They alter the normal functions of these cells and force them into making more viruses, usually destroying the host cells when this process is completed. Sometimes the tissue damage is irreparable. Examples include the cells of the nervous system invaded by poliovirus, or the abnormalities that can occur in the developing tissues of a foetus carried in the womb of a woman who contracts rubella infection during the early weeks of pregnancy. Vaccines still represent our best chance of preventing such things from happening.

Vaccination is now part of our way of life. Most of us have little say in the matter because our parents take us to receive the recommended courses of childhood immunisations before our formative years. During adulthood we may require vaccinations appropriate to our employment, sometimes before travelling to foreign countries, or when we become older and more vulnerable to infections such as influenza. The benefits to Man's well-being have been immeasurable. In the western world, many potentially fatal infections that decimated our forebears are now held in check and we take an ever-increasing life expectancy for granted. One of the major causes of death or disfigurement, smallpox, has been eradicated from the globe. The dreadful statistics of child mortality in Victorian times arising from the effects of infectious diseases, coupled with the debilitating effects of malnutrition, are now only recorded in some third world countries. When a threat from a new virus emerges this immediately stimulates research into the development of a vaccine. Sometimes this can prove an extremely difficult task. We are still awaiting an effective vaccine to stem the rising tide of the Human Immunodeficiency Virus, despite the massive research effort under way in many countries around the globe. The introduction of MenC vaccine in 1999 brought a reduction of over 80% in the type C form of meningitis, but there is no vaccination yet available against a related species of the bacterium (*Neisseria meningitidis* type B) which is also responsible for this medical condition. Solving this problem remains a priority for British researchers because Meningitis B has always been more common in the UK. Thankfully, infection with another bacterium associated with meningitis, *Haemophilus influenzae*, can now be thwarted by immunisation with Hib vaccine.

Modern technologies have brought safer and more effective vaccines. At the time of writing there is news of a better formulation designed to enhance immunity to tuberculosis. The clinical trials are timely - TB is one of several diseases that have staged a comeback in recent years. There are new and exciting developments in progress. A vaccine to prevent infection by the Human Papilloma Virus has just been licensed. Results from trials look impressive and this 'jab' is likely to bring a significant reduction in the incidence of cervical cancer. It is estimated that one malnourished child dies every minute from dehydration caused by Rotavirus associated diarrhoea. A clinical trial of a Rotavirus vaccine has begun in Mexico. Let us hope this will fare better than two previous Rotavirus vaccines that were withdrawn during former trials. Other candidate vaccines under investigation at present include those directed against Herpesvirus and malaria. The current policy for routine childhood multivalent vaccines is to increase the number of components so these stimulate immunity to more microbes in one jab. Thus the 'triple' vaccine of old has now become 'quintuple', and contains diphtheria, tetanus, whooping cough, polio and Hib. A great deal of research is being conducted in the groundbreaking science of DNA vaccines. These have potential applications in the treatment of some non-infectious conditions such as B cell lymphoma, myeloma and other leukaemias, but it is too early to know what benefits this approach will yield.

The introduction of new vaccines has sometimes been accompanied by controversy. A report published in a leading medical journal during February 1998 caused some parents great concern over the Measles, Mumps, Rubella vaccine (MMR). It would be inappropriate to discuss this in detail here, but suffice to say that circumstances unknown to the editors at the time would have resulted in rejection of the manuscript, had they been disclosed. Public confidence in the British health authorities was already in decline after the government issued conflicting statements on 'mad cow disease'. This was then further damaged by populist hype of a flawed MMR investigation that should never have been published. Problems arose from the huge media coverage, together with some irresponsible reportage, leading to an understandable loss of assurance in the minds of anxious parents who were trying to make sense of an unnecessary debate.

Such controversies may lead to a reduction in the uptake of a besmirched vaccine. When this happens over a period of time there is a loss of 'herd immunity' in the population as a whole. Public health authorities are able to calculate the percentage of individuals with vaccine-induced immunity that is required to prevent outbreaks of infectious diseases in the community. If the percentage falls below its recommended level, there is always a rise in the incidence of the disease in question. This has occurred in some areas where the number of MMR jabs fell below critical limits and the result has been a considerable increase in the prevalence of mumps. Similar consequences have been observed before, when other vaccines have been in the headlines. The only exception to this delicate equation is the non-requirement of vaccination when an infectious disease has been completely eliminated. At present, humanity's score in this respect is just one. Smallpox was officially declared eradicated from the world in 1979.

Our relationship with microbes is complex. Some are essential components of our biological function, others may be harmful and even life threatening. Our natural inclination to view pathogenic viruses, bacteria and parasites solely as agents which cause us disease leaves us with an overly simplistic appreciation of the process. Routes to infection are not unidirectional. The real situation is that we are participants in an intricate *ménage a trois*. To understand how our bodies become victims of microbial invasion we must take the natures of both microbe and human host into account, together with the circumstances pertaining at the time.

These three factors are always relevant, and are weighted singly or in combination. Each of the segments of this triangle of aetiology may be subject to variation to a greater or lesser extent. For instance, HIV is able to override our defences because it is able to undergo multiple mutations. Some people suffer infections such as chickenpox more severely than others because they have immune systems that are impaired through predisposing medical conditions. Man can be his own worst enemy. The emergence of a growing number of multi-resistant bacteria has been caused by unrestricted public access to antibiotics, their clinical over-prescription, and a clandestine misuse in agriculture. Methicillin Resistant *Staphylococcus aureus* (MRSA) is just one example. Contrary to what our politicians tell us, the unacceptable prevalence of MRSA in our hospitals has little to do with the cleanliness of wards but everything to do with the people who inhabit them. Countries such as Japan and the USA have excellent reputations for clean hospitals but are still beset by MRSA. The way forward has been demonstrated by the Netherlands, where detection and treatment of healthy human carriers, together with a rigid adherence to intelligent infection control policies, has virtually eliminated the problems associated with this troublesome bacterium.

Sometimes a combination of factors may result in the emergence of new threats such as 'bird flu', and Severe Acute Respiratory Syndrome (SARS). Viruses of animals or birds may jump the species barrier into humans, especially in areas of widespread co-habitation as in the Far East. Coupling the resultant evolution of a potentially dangerous respiratory virus with the present day necessity for widespread and frequent air travel creates the ideal conditions for a pandemic i.e. a rapid world-wide spread of a disease against which we have no protection. Changes in man's social behaviour may also prove a significant factor in our vulnerability to pathogenic organisms, and this can work either way. Improvements in diet and housing conditions had brought a reduction in the prevalence of tuberculosis even before the advent of streptomycin. In contrast, when the newfound carnal freedoms of the rock n roll era gave way to the totally permissive society of the 'Swinging Sixties' there was a noticeable rise in Herpesvirus, Chlamydial and other sexually transmitted diseases.

When manning the barricades we need to recognise situations where vaccination is not practicable - or in some cases, must be avoided at all costs. The Englishman continues to suffer 'his usual bloody cold' because it is not yet possible to manufacture a single vaccine which will stimulate immunity to more than 120 strains of common cold virus. When a new type of influenza virus emerges, through inter-species transfer and mutation, the existing vaccines are usually ineffective and it takes time to manufacture one for appropriate deployment. These problems will only be solved when new vaccine technologies or chemotherapies are developed, and it will be interesting to see if the research announced recently will prove an effective long-term strategy against influenza in the future.

Nutrition is an essential factor in optimising responses to vaccination. Human immune mechanisms need a constant power supply, and are fuelled by energy obtained from the nourishment of normal life support. A severely malnourished third-world child will succumb to vaccine-preventable diseases because its body has already directed limited resources towards an effort to survive. Global vaccine efficiency will only be achieved if our world is fed adequately.

Occasionally, there are times when vaccination would be harmful; all licensed vaccines have instructions for contra-indication, which list the circumstances when they should not be used. Pregnancy is just one example.

Members of the public became more concerned about the potential hazards that appeared to be associated with vaccination as the incidence of once common infections such as diphtheria and whooping cough declined. I would be misleading the reader if I appear to dismiss any element of risk. There is no such thing as a 'perfect' vaccine that protects everyone who receives it and is entirely safe, but the risk is latent and is usually associated with a lack of tolerance in the recipient. Most side effects are mild. The occasional serious reaction is nearly always an unrelated event which has happened by co-incidence. There is always a theoretical risk to us when any medical procedure is employed on our behalf, ranging from surgery to the simple act of swallowing a couple of aspirin tablets. Most of us accept this and put it into perspective, as with many things. There is a danger in crossing the road or driving a car, but we follow the advice in the Highway Code and the risk is part of our everyday lives. Worries created by irresponsible scare stories in the media must not be given the same credence as proven scientific facts. Medicine is the most demanding of disciplines. New vaccines are subjected to very extensive and rigorous programmes of evaluation before being licensed in Britain or the USA, and there is a wealth of information available to the public from national and local health authorities.

Vaccines are here to stay for the foreseeable future because there are no viable alternatives at the present time. They have played a major part in reducing infectious diseases to an all time low. In our fight against an unseen, ubiquitous and ever-changing microbial adversary, vaccination has become a social responsibility. We ignore this at our peril. Humans believe their species has evolved to become the dominant life form on this planet, but they should be aware that their ability to control microbes is limited. The worst consequences of infection can be disastrous, either internationally or at a personal level. The next chapter includes a harrowing glimpse of an event which occurred less than seventy years ago, and is an example of the tragedies that can befall the unprotected.

Chapter 2

Yesterday's Witness

The origins of vaccination are inextricably linked with one highly dangerous virus disease - smallpox. The biology and history of this most devastating of mankind's afflictions has been set down in many fine volumes which are readily accessible, and it is neither feasible nor necessary to provide more than an overview in this book. However, I have tried to bring a fresh approach to the second half of this chapter, so that the reader is confronted with the horror of smallpox in everyday human terms.

The smallpox virus is the largest and the most complex of the human viruses, but much smaller in size than a bacterium. It measures 300 millionths of a millimeter in length, and is brick shaped. Details of its structure are only seen when the virus is viewed under an electron microscope. Smallpox disease is thought to have originated in North-East Africa c10,000 BC when hunter gatherers turned to agriculture and began to settle in communities. The earliest clinical evidence is the presence of typical skin lesions on the faces of Egyptian mummies of the 18th and 20th Dynasties. These include Pharaoh Rameses V who died in 1157 BC. The first clinical description of symptoms was written by the Persian physician, Rhazes, in 910 AD. It is thought that the disease may have been carried to the East by Egyptian merchants, then spread throughout North Africa and the Mediterranean during the 6th- 8th centuries by Arab invaders. Outbreaks began to appear in Europe when the crusaders returned from the wars in the Levant. Smallpox was introduced into the New World by the conquistadors and it spread like wildfire. The population of Mexico numbered 25 million when the Spanish arrived in 1518 and was reduced to only 1.6 million within a hundred years.

By the sixteenth century the disease had become established in Britain. Queen Elizabeth I survived an attack at the age of 29 in 1562 but she was only one of many monarchs to suffer. The virus was no respecter of rank or position. Smallpox proliferated among princes and peasants throughout the European countries in the following 200 years, killing about 400,000 people annually. Macaulay, writing in 1694 about the death of Queen Mary II, noted that smallpox had become more prevalent than the plague:

'The havoc of the plague had been far more rapid: but the plague had visited our shores only once or twice within living memory; and the smallpox was always present, filling the churchyards with corpses, tormenting with constant fears all whom it had not yet stricken, leaving on those whose lives it spared the hideous traces of its power, turning the babe into a changeling at which the mother shuddered, and making the eyes and cheeks of the betrothed maiden objects of horror to the lover'.

Fatal victims included six members of the Stuart dynasty, among them William the 11-year-old son of Queen Anne. The resulting constitutional crisis led to the Act of Settlement of 1701, which prevented any claim to the throne from the Catholic descendants of James II. Thus, a tiny pathogenic virus was a factor in bringing the House of Hanover to rule over a Protestant England.

Smallpox was responsible for more than one third of all blindness. In urban centres like London it was assumed that nearly everyone would contract the disease during their lives, but this usually happened when they were young. Those who lived bore scars of the pocks thereafter. Voltaire survived, as did Mozart, George Washington, Abraham Lincoln and Joseph Stalin. Stalin would not permit un-retouched photographs of his scarred face to be published during his early years of power.

Various clinical forms of the infection existed. The most virulent was *Variola major*, with case fatality rates ranging from 20% – 98%. Patients developed a high fever, with rigors and prostration, often accompanied by nausea and vomiting. The fever relented after about four days and a rash would appear over the body. Maculopapular lesions preceded vesicles, then pustules, which dried into scabs that fell off after a few weeks. At the same time, the virus was also wreaking havoc in the tissues of internal organs. Patients with fulminating smallpox developed mucocutaneous haemorrhages before the skin lesions appeared. Malignant and benign versions were also clinically differentiated. Modified smallpox was a benign type and could occur in vaccinated persons. This included *Variola sine eruptione*, when the patient did not have a rash. Another less virulent form of the disease, which caused a mild form of smallpox with a case fatality rate of only 0.5% - 2%, was known as *Variola minor*. This was endemic in Africa and South America.

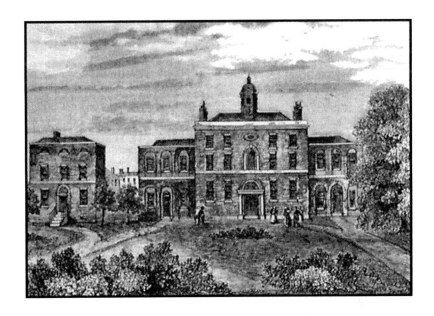

The London Smallpox Hospital as it looked in 1800.
This was situated at the end of Euston Road but the building no longer exists.
The present Kings Cross Railway Station was built on the site in 1851 - 52.

Smallpox was a major problem in 31 countries as recently as 35 years ago, with a total of 10 – 15 million new cases of infection each year. The annual mortality from the disease was more than 2 million. It is thought that smallpox killed at least one billion of the world's population in the one hundred years that preceded its eradication.

Quoting mortality figures and historical records is horrifying enough, but the reality of this disease is brought into sharpest focus when viewed in the context of the family. I have been exceptionally privileged to talk about this with a late friend who was a survivor of the infection. What follows is a harrowing account, given by a man whose family was destroyed by smallpox, and is typical of the sufferings of countless millions of families throughout history. The names have been changed but this edited transcript of a taped interview conducted on the 9th December 2002 is otherwise unaltered. This story is related by a 68-year-old man reaching back in his mind to an event which took place 62 years earlier. What follows is expressed in his own words:

'I was born in Lahore in 1934, that was before Partition of course, but this happened when I was about five or six. It happened in Calcutta I would think, because Dad was serving in His Majesty's Forces. He was an RAMC operating theatre assistant. We lived in a compound of army quarters. Army families were billeted out of the city. This was India just before the war (WW2), and of course we had servants and people like that.

Relatives are very vague in my memory but I can remember my grandfather. He was out in India with the telegraph communications. I can remember my brothers and sisters of course. Elaine was the oldest, Vivian was next, then came Leonard, then Maria, next was me, and then Molly who was the youngest. Dad was immunised against smallpox because the British Forces had to be immunised, and as far as I know, he was the only vaccinated person in the family.

The medical facilities were basic at that time. There was no GP as such. In those days, hospitalisation was done mainly for His Majesty's Forces and Europeans and the like. Hospitals were comprised of the basic army facilities in the field. There weren't a lot of staff around, like nursing staff. I don't remember people like sisters and matrons. Dad was providing some medical help for the local community. I don't know how he was keeping himself financially solvent.

Hygiene was very limited. All the time in the (army) centre, it was kept well controlled, but as soon as you started to move from that particular area you were out in the open. You were out to the world, exposed to anything. Dysentery was very prominent. That's how it started with me. I think I was the perpetrator of it (the smallpox). I was told afterwards that I had brought it in to the family. There must have been a lot of people going down with it because it hit that part of India badly. The infection could have been carried by anybody.

It was very hot, perhaps July or August. I had dysentery and a fever, and my throat was drying up. I wanted something to drink. That's when Elaine and one or two of the others wanted to nurse me and that sort of thing. After that it turned different. My throat started to swell up, then the others fell down with it, either Maria or Elaine, then after that it came down very quickly. They realised what it was – something very contagious. I started getting a few skin lesions then. My throat was very sore – everywhere was itching so badly and I wanted to scratch, so they tied my hands together.

They realised what was happening. I had started with dysentery, a temperature as well, then I was materialising with the spots – they looked a mauve colour and were full of pus – they irritated very much. Then my mother went down with it. I could feel the tension in Dad's voice. That's when they moved everybody. The whole family was in one particular 'pest house' as they would call them. They weren't stone buildings, they were prefabricated, shuttered, and kept purely for isolation. It was just like a Nissen hut, with the windows and doors locked. They had padlocks and chains on both doors. We were all on our own – the whole family. After being cut off, we didn't know much about what was happening outside the building.

Dad was doing lots of the nursing himself. In those days, iodine was the main disinfectant and I could smell the iodine. They had put a small dilution on my spots to see if they could do something. I can smell that iodine now.

Dad and another nurse looked after us and that was it. I never saw anybody being moved. I can remember my mother going through it quite drastically, Bless her, even to the stage where she would ask Dad for water. She would say 'my throat's so dry, please give me some.' The others were there. I can remember voices coming through – I must have gone delirious – I can remember voices in the background. I don't know what happened. A curtain came down then, just like that.....

(Within two weeks after contracting smallpox, only the father and two of his children survived out of a family of eight).

After the annihilation of my family I was sent to Dehra Dun to convalesce at my grandfather's place. My grandmother was dead by then and I don't know where Molly went. I noticed about the others. I wondered where they were. All that was said was they would follow up. They kept it away from me till a later stage. Dad went through a traumatic stage. Twice, he nearly killed himself – that's what I was told afterwards. We had a manservant. I think it was him that stopped Dad committing suicide. After my father was de-mobbed he took up a position with Spencers & Co. They were well known throughout India. He used to work up in Simla. I remember the semi-Victorian buildings and the verandahs. It was very regal. I wonder if people realize how grand those buildings were. Then Molly and I were sent to boarding school.

I left India in 1946, when we had Partition. Dad said everyone must go, because the Foreign Office said all Europeans living in India should get out quickly. All three of us came over on the Johan Van Oldenbarnevelt, a Dutch liner used as an Allied troopship. I then resumed my schooling in England.'

The man who spoke these words died about thirty months after I talked with him. He had approved the transcript and agreed to its publication. Medical textbooks contain clinical descriptions and photographs of cases, but rarely the personal recollections of patients who survived the disease. My friend's interview is set down in this book because nobody will have had experience of smallpox infection in the future. His account has now become part of the historical record.

This was the tragedy of one family amongst millions of others who suffered similar experiences over a timescale reaching back to the distant mists of antiquity. Man must have felt under siege from the beginning. It was little wonder that he looked for a means to defend himself against what Macaulay termed, 'the most terrible of all the ministers of death'. The battle started in the Far East, in unknown lands where knowledge of the peoples was scant to those in the West. Men and women began to fight back against their invisible foe. As the news of their progress travelled slowly across Asia towards the Mediterranean, smallpox was already sowing the seeds of its own destruction, for the early methods of protection involved use of the disease itself. A decade into the eighteenth century, the European stage was set - but it was a woman who took the leading role in Act One - and this was at a time when convention decreed that the cast should be exclusively male.

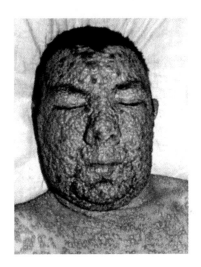

A case of benign smallpox at Halifax, England, in March 1953 showing the clinical appearance on the 9th day of the rash with swelling of the facial tissues. Skin lesions are usually confluent on the head, as seen here, and at other extremities of the body. The patient survived.

Chapter 3

Lady Mary's Pomatum

It was a hot August afternoon in the year 1713. The turnpike keeper waved the travellers away, mopped his brow, and returned to doze in the welcome shade of a tree. The coach continued on its journey, rattling and bumping along a rutted highway that snaked through the countryside southwest of London. Jolted unmercifully within the coach sat Lady Mary Pierrepoint, the 24 year-old daughter of the Earl of Kingston. She gazed out of the window at an uncertain future, but must have felt confident that she had made the right decision. Her situation was becoming intolerable. Spurning convention, she had resorted to desperate measures. Lady Mary was fleeing to escape an unsolicited marriage arranged by her father, a capricious widower and rake who had often placed responsibility for running the household on his daughter's young shoulders. Her destination was an inn, where she planned to meet and elope with her close friend, the resourceful Edward Wortley Montagu. They had known each other for about seven years and their long courtship had progressed in tandem with a correspondence of increasing fervour. Lady Mary was not in love with Wortley Montagu and had considerable misgivings, but saw the elopement as an infinitely preferable alternative to marrying into 'Hell' with Clotworthy Skeffington – her father's choice. On reaching the inn, which was situated somewhere along the present A30 road, Lady Mary retired early and consequently failed to see Edward who was searching the premises for her. His prowling led the clientele to suspect him of being a highwayman! Next morning she continued to one of the family properties, West Dean in Wiltshire, where Edward came to rescue her a few days later. They were married at Salisbury on the 23rd August.

Wortley Montagu was a self made man and a member of parliament who had progressed to prominence in the Whig party through his own efforts. He was given a position of responsibility in the Treasury. The couple entered London society and they were invited to attend court.

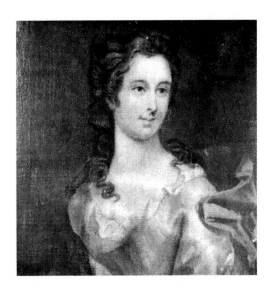

Lady Mary Wortley Montagu, from an oil portrait by C F Zincke
Wellcome Library, London.

Lady Mary was an exceptional woman - very intelligent and literate but also regarded as one of the great beauties of her time. She was a gifted writer, the authoress of many satirical essays on society, politics, women's issues and rights denied to women. Other works included accounts of her travels, poetry and much correspondence. She was competent in Latin, French, Italian and Turkish. Her contemporaries were the leading literary figures of the early eighteenth century. Born way ahead of her time, she suffered the difficulties of being an accomplished woman in the exclusive realm of a man's world. Her life is the subject of a magnificent biography by Isobel Grundy.

Lady Mary's brother died from smallpox in 1713. Two years later, in the month of December, she contracted the dread disease herself and was fighting for her life. She recovered after being close to death and was facially scarred. The loss of her eyelashes marred Lady Mary's good looks. Not impressed with the dubious abilities of the medical profession in their attempts to effect a cure, she wrote a rather heartfelt poem entitled

'Saturday - The Small-pox. Flavia'. Four lines from this poem give a clue to the motivation for her actions three years later:

'Ye cruel chemists, what withheld your aid?
Could no pomatum save a trembling maid?
How false and trifling is that art ye boast
No art can give me back my beauty lost'

In 1716 Edward was appointed as the British Ambassador to Turkey. To reach this destination they both travelled overland to Constantinople, which took them from August until January the following year. Many considered it unthinkable that a woman would attempt to undertake such an arduous journey, but Lady Mary did so, and described her experiences in detailed letters. When she arrived in Constantinople Lady Mary explored many aspects of an alien culture that was previously unknown to English women. She visited mosques in disguise and was invited to meet the Sultan. He allowed her to enter the harem to talk to those installed as his wives and concubines. Most noteworthy of Lady Mary's experiences during her stay in Turkey was her observation of the technique used by elderly female practitioners for protecting the young against smallpox. Where had this strange medicine originated?

There must have been a moment, now lost in the mists of antiquity, when someone noticed that the survivors of some types of pestilences appeared to possess a magical protection against further such afflictions. One of the earliest records was set down in 430 BC by the Athenian general, Thucydides, writing about a plague during the war with Sparta:

'...yet the ones who felt most pity for the sick were those who had the plague themselves and recovered from it. They knew what it was like and at the same time felt themselves to be safe, for no-one caught the disease twice, or if he did, the second attack was never fatal'.

Common experiences over a period of time must have helped to evolve the concept into a traditional belief. This preceded a giant leap for mankind when an unknown sage supposed that actually giving someone a tiny morsel of a disease might have the same protective effect as a natural infection. By accident or design, this happened with smallpox. Knowledge of the Chinese technique of insufflation had reached the fringe of the western world by 1000 AD. Dried smallpox scabs were ground into powder and this was blown into the nose of a recipient through a hollow pipe, rather like using a peashooter. Another way of achieving the same result was to dip a fragment of cotton into a ripe smallpox pustule, allow it to dry, then place it into the patient's nostrils. The Persians preferred to ingest powdered scabs, but the Greeks and Turks developed a method of introducing live smallpox material into a small wound in the skin. Today this is referred to as variolation (*Variola* is the scientific name for the smallpox virus) but Lady Mary referred to the practice as 'ingrafting'. An extract from a letter to her friend, Lady Sarah Chiswell, contains a description of the technique:

'Apropos of distempers, I am going to tell you a thing that will make you wish yourself here. The small-pox so fatal and so general amongst us, is here entirely harmless, by the invention of ingrafting, which is the term they give it. There is a set of old women, who make it their business to perform the operation. People make parties for the purpose, and when they are met, the old woman comes with a nutshell full of the matter of the best sort of small-pox, and asks you what vein you please to have opened. She immediately rips open that you offer her with a large needle and puts into the vein as much matter as can lay upon the head of her needle, and after that binds up the little wound; and in this manner opens four or five veins. Every year thousands undergo this operation; they take the small-pox here by way of diversion, as they take the waters in other countries. I am patriot enough to take pains to bring this useful invention into fashion in England; and I should not fail to write to some of our doctors very particularly about it, if I knew any one of them that I thought had virtue enough to destroy such a considerable branch of their revenue for the good of mankind ...Perhaps, if I live to return, I may, however have courage to war with them'.

It is very unlikely that the 'old woman' opened veins, as the aim was to induce a localized smallpox infection, and this would have been achieved more effectively by making superficial (cutaneous) incisions.

The earliest news of Chinese intranasal techniques was communicated to Dr Martin Lister in 1700 by a trader working for the East India Company. Lister was a Fellow of the Royal Society but his information failed to excite interest and no action was taken. Variolation had been introduced into the Ottoman Empire around 1670 by Circassian traders. The Turkish practice observed by Lady Mary had already been reported to the Royal Society, in a letter dated December 1713, by a physician named Emanuel Timoni who was living in Constantinople. The letter was summarised in the Society's journal. Timoni (FRS) had acquired his medical qualifications in Padua but also possessed a degree from Oxford. His account stimulated discussion and a motion was agreed, instructing the secretary to obtain further information. Two years later, the Royal Society published a more extensive description written by Dr Giacomo Pylarini, who was serving as the British Consul in Smyrna. The British medical establishment must have seen little merit in the reports. Despite widespread publicity, they did not appear to adopt the technique, although smallpox was a constant problem in Britain. Presumably, the physicians were unwilling to risk their reputations (and lucrative vocations) by adopting this novel idea.

During the spring of 1718 Lady Mary made a momentous decision - one which would influence a change in the passive attitude holding sway in Britain. Whilst her husband was away on official duties she requested that her five-year-old son Edward be protected against smallpox by ingrafting. Presumably motivated by her own bitter experience of the disease and its fatal outcome in her brother, Lady Mary was practising the new philosophy of the Enlightenment Movement which she had adopted with enthusiasm. Suffering and hardship were no longer assumed to be pre-ordained - and therefore endured - but might be alleviated by Man's intervention if this was deemed possible. Perhaps Montagu felt she had stumbled upon an effective 'pomatum' by serendipity. Lady Mary appears to have taken sole responsibility for the decision, though she may have discussed it with Timoni who was now a part-time diplomat and her family physician. The project received active support from the embassy surgeon, Charles Maitland, and on the 18th March they summoned an elderly nurse who was well known in Constantinople for her ingrafting expertise. The nurse pricked the boy's arm with a rusty needle and applied some smallpox matter to the puncture. Maitland repeated the procedure on the second arm 'with my own instrument' and covered the lesions with dressings. About a hundred spots appeared over Edward Jnr's body after a few days. These quickly became crusts which dropped off leaving no trace, though marks of the wounds would have remained at the sites of ingrafting. The Rev Crosse, who was chaplain of the embassy, preached vehemently against this incident.

The Wortley Montagus set sail for home later the same year. Their slow voyage on the *Preston* was uneventful but they took time to visit a number of Mediterranean antiquities which provided interesting diversions. The parents disembarked at Genoa and set out overland for England, leaving son and daughter to continue their sea journey in the company of an Armenian nurse. The family was finally re-united at home in the New Year and settled down once more to the proprieties of the London social scene.

Lady Mary's preoccupations with her literary contemporaries, approaches by extra-marital suitors, and an ill-advised speculation in the South Sea Company, were short-lived. Early in 1721 smallpox re-surfaced in London with a vengeance. By April the death toll was occupying ever-increasing space in the obituary columns and had brought formal visiting to a standstill. There was heated debate amongst factions of the medical profession about the treatment of cases, but no consideration of how the pestilence might be prevented. Lady Mary took matters into her own hands once again. She contacted Charles Maitland again and asked him to use ingrafting to protect her three-year-old daughter Mary. He was wary - conscious of his professional standing. Undertaking the deliberate infection of a healthy child with potentially lethal disease could bring him into disrepute. This was the City of London, vastly different to a distant capital at the Golden Horn which many considered to be at the border of civilisation. Maitland insisted he should be attended by some medical witnesses who could testify that he had acted in an honourable manner.

According to Lady Louisa Smart, three learned doctors from the College of Physicians were nominated by the government. Maitland obtained material from a smallpox patient who was not severely affected. He carried out the procedure as before, using both of the child's arms. Daughter Mary was closely monitored by the official observers. She developed a fever at ten days, followed by the emergence of pocks. After a total of three weeks she had returned to normal health. The event generated considerable interest. News was communicated within medical circles and discussed widely among the upper echelons of society by friends of the Wortley Montagus. People referred to this revolutionary development as 'The Inoculation'. The terminology passed into common parlance. Inoculation soon became the subject of a heated debate between doctors, journalists and the clergy, similar to the modern day attitudes that sometimes give rise to dispute over new advances in science or medicine.

Word now reached the ear of royalty. Caroline, Princess of Wales, was very interested in science and supported Lady Mary over the inoculation issue. One of her own children had nearly died of smallpox. She encouraged some physicians to petition George I for his patronage of an experiment to demonstrate the effectiveness of inoculation. Six condemned convicts from Newgate Prison, three of each sex, volunteered for The Royal Experiment which took place on the 9th August 1721 amid considerable comment and attention from the press. Maitland sought professional backing from Edward Tarry, a doctor with Turkish experience. The convicts were inoculated in the presence of a large group of eminent witnesses. Five of the volunteers (the sixth admitted to having had smallpox previously) exhibited a brief but mild illness and then recovered. They were all pardoned and released from prison. One of the women was instructed to share a bed with a young boy who was suffering from smallpox in order to prove her immunity – she was unaffected.

Inoculation became the lead topic in every newspaper, each expressing a different opinion. The Royal Society was gradually won round. The President of the College of Physicians, Sir Hans Sloane, had his grandchildren inoculated. Princess Caroline persuaded Maitland to inoculate two of her daughters. After a slow start, the practice was accepted by Lady Mary's friends and relations, together with those who had reason to fear disease through personal experience. Others saw a way to make money. The new *modus operandi* was gradually taken up by doctors, apothecaries, and even by some who had no previous connection with the medical profession at all. Hostile opposition came mostly from a vociferous clergy. The Rev Edmund Massey delivered a sermon on 8th July 1722 at St Andrews, Holborn, entitled *'The Dangerous and Sinful Practice of Inoculation'*. There were also those with a political axe to grind. William Wagstaffe leapt into print, protesting that:

'Posterity will scarcely be brought to believe, that an Experiment practised only by a few Ignorant Women, amongst an illiterate and unthinking people[*], shou'd on a sudden, and upon a slender experience, so far obtain in one of the Politest Nations in the World, as to be received into the Royal Palace'
([*] Wagstaffe's opinion of the Turks)

Lady Mary sought to counter this rhetoric by writing 'A Plain Account of the Innoculating of the Small Pox', published in the *Flying-Post* on the 13th September 1722. Some of the problems were caused by practitioners who had altered and complicated the Turkish technique, presumably in order to increase their fees. Recipients were obliged to prepare for inoculation by following a meagre low-protein vegetable diet for some weeks, and were bled several times during this period. Vomiting and purging were induced by the administration of a mercurial compound. The unfortunate patients received the inoculation in this thoroughly weakened state. One or more deep incisions were opened with a lancet, and the live smallpox material applied to the wounds. Lady Mary knew that all of this was absolute nonsense and said as much in her *Flying-Post* essay. No preparation, a small laceration with a needle, and a minute amount of smallpox inoculum was the method perfected by the Turks, but an exclusive and male dominated medical establishment was certainly not going to take any notice of a mere woman bringing this to their attention.

By the 1740s inoculation had become established among the gentry in Britain. It never achieved popularity with the general public, although figures compiled by the observant Secretary to the Royal Society

(James Jurin) showed that the measures worked to some extent. There were always problems - occasions when inoculation resulted in illness or death. The most significant drawback was that inoculation could spread smallpox into areas of the country where it had been quiescent. The poor looked upon inoculators with mistrust and were sometimes encouraged to submit to treatment by being paid. In the spring of 1722 ten people received a total of £4-9-0 from the Yetminster Vestry for complying. However, opinions differed greatly, and other local authorities would have none of it. An extract dated January 11th 1786 from a minute book of the Lytchett Minster Vestry, stored in the Dorset Archives, reads as follows:

'We the Inhabitants of Lytchett Minster Being met for Vestry Conserning the Ease of The poor and allso We do agree if aney person or Persons Shall or do Bring or ofer to Bring Aney Distemper Sutch as Cald the Small pox Shall Be prosecuted by the parish Offesis acording to law And it is farther agreed that no person or persons Shall Bring the Small pox into the parish by Enocklashon'

Some enthusiasts did recognise the inherent dangers of inoculation and made suitable provision for the isolation of those undergoing the procedure. There is unique evidence of this hidden away in a forested area of West Sussex, near Chichester, and described by Francis Steer in The Lancet in 1956. During the mid-eighteenth century, a local landowner, Sir James Peachey of West Dean, built a small cottage to be used as an isolation hospital for members of his family and his estate workers who were receiving inoculation. This brick and flint building is entered as 'Black Bushe' in some Deeds of 1741. Now much altered, it still stands on the wooded ridge which runs northwards from Bow Hill, some two and a half kilometres from the nearest village, and is accessed only by a rough track. Patients remained here until they were considered safe to be returned to their homes and families. Within the now modernised cottage are two of the original internal doors, constructed of deal and darkened with age. They are covered with finely carved inscriptions of names and dates, providing a record of those who were incarcerated. The dates of these testimonies range from 1753 to 1788.

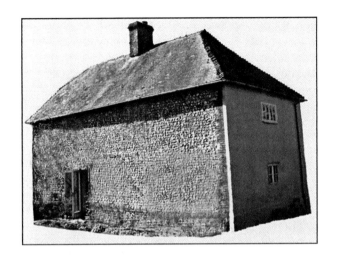

Photo-reconstruction of how Black Bushe House appeared in the 1950s. The east facing wall had no windows. The siting of windows in the 1700s is unknown.

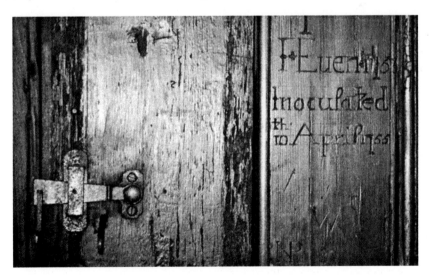

One of the many inscriptions on the original doors inside Black Bushe House. 'I Euen Inoculated 10th April 1755'

The example in the illustration shows the quality of the carving, and reads, *I Euen Inoculated 10th April 1755*. An examination of the local burial records suggests that none of the patients died during their stay, but Sir James's isolation hospital represents a sensible precaution of containment.

Inoculation continued into the early 1800s. Some practitioners were more successful than others in what became a competitive business environment. One example of a typical advertisement for such services can be found in the Salisbury and Winchester Journal for the 29th January 1776, and is shown here in a format which is similar to the original.

SUTTONIAN Art of INOCULATION

Rolfe and Hargraves most respectfully
inform the public, that they have taken and opened
a house near HINDON, for the reception of Patients in
Inoculation, commonly called FONTHILL-LODGE; which
has been many years made use of by Mr. Spencer for that
purpose, and well known for the healthiness and pleasant-
ness of its situation.

Patients are provided with every necessary accommodation (tea, sugar, and linen excepted) from two to three
guineas, according to the different accommodations required
under the immediate inspection of Mrs. Rolfe, and not left
to the care of servants.

Mrs. Rolfe, late Mrs. Hargraves, was several years house-
keeper to the celebrated Dr Sutton, and by assisting him in
his business she acquired the perfect art and mystery, now
called the Suttonian method of Inoculation, both in respect
to the practice and the composition of his medicines.

Mr. Spencer takes the liberty to request of his friends and
customers the continuance of their favours to Mess. Rolfe
and Hargraves.

The renowned Dr Robert Sutton began his work in Suffolk in 1757, and made a very good living by using a simplified technique based on the Turkish version which had been advocated by Lady Mary. He advertised '*A new method of Inoculating for the Small Pox*' in the Ipswich

Journal on the 1st May 1762, but he was careful to keep the intricacies of his method a closely guarded secret. His son Daniel did not publish full details until 1796, so it is unlikely that the enterprising Mrs Rolfe had acquired the 'perfect art and mystery' in its totality.

Inoculation was first used in America in 1721. Though this coincided with Maitland's second application of the procedure in London, the same technique was introduced in the New World quite independently of the happenings in Europe. The Rev Cotton Mather of Boston was told about the practice by his slave, Onesimus, who had come from South-Western Libya in North Africa. His story was confirmed by other Africans and slave traders. Mather then read Timoni's report, but was unaware of Maitland's inoculation of Lady Mary's son in 1718. When an outbreak of smallpox spread throughout Boston in the spring of 1721, Mather wrote to all the physicians in the city and encouraged them to inoculate as a means of containing the disease. Only Zabdiel Boylston responded at first. He began inoculating despite opposition from his colleagues and physical abuse from some of the townsfolk. A hand grenade was thrown through a window of Mather's house but fortunately it did not explode. Boylston slowly gathered a little support, and by the following year, showed figures which gave a mortality rate of 2.5% among 242 inoculated persons, compared with one of 15% of those dying among 5889 cases of natural smallpox. The Boston authorities placed inoculation under official control in May 1722, and Boylston had to promise not to proceed any further without approval. However, these events in Boston could be said to have marked the beginnings of preventive measures against infectious disease in the United States.

Lady Mary parted from Edward in 1739 to live the rest of her life abroad in Italy and France, returning to London in 1762, the year after her husband died. Soon after her return she fell ill with breast cancer and died aged 73 on the 21st August the same year. She didn't find the pomatum that she sought from the medical fraternity but it may be argued that she saved many lives through her influence and determination. One of her great nieces erected a memorial to her in 1789. This may be seen on a wall just inside the entrance of Lichfield Cathedral.

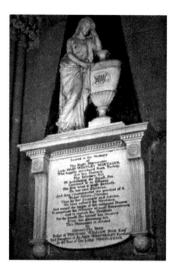

The memorial plaque to Lady Mary Wortley Montagu set up in Lichfield Cathedral by a great niece in 1789.

In 1793 the Chester physician, John Haygarth (surely the forerunner of that rare and valuable breed, The Consultant in Infectious Diseases) suggested that smallpox could be eliminated from Britain if widespread inoculation was supported by the isolation of infected persons, backed by a policy of incentives and penalties. He was 184 years ahead of his time. The global eradication of smallpox was to be achieved far into the future by employing a similar approach, but with vaccination as the means of stimulating immunity.

Inoculation did offer a form of protection against the ravages of Dryden's 'Foul Disease' when performed correctly, though its application was always potentially hazardous. The practice only ceased completely when vaccination gained acceptance by a hesitant medical profession at the beginning of the 19th Century. In Act 2 of Goldsmith's *'She Stoops to Conquer'* Mrs Hardcastle exclaims, 'I vow, since inoculation began, there is no such thing to be seen as a plain woman.' I am sure that Lady Mary would have been delighted! Despite bigoted and chauvinistic opposition, her audacity and determination had made an effective contribution to the progress of medicine, but she could never have imagined that her actions would help to provide the foundation of what was to follow.

Chapter 4

Benjamin Jesty – The First Vaccinator

By 1774 George III had been on the English throne for fourteen years. 'Farmer George' and his Prime Minister, Lord North, were preoccupied with the troublesome colonists in America. During December the previous year, the self styled 'Sons of Liberty' had emptied a consignment of tea into the harbour at Boston in protest at the British Government's plans to impose a tea duty. Now the upstarts had petitioned for the removal of their governor-general! North's parliament was imposing four Coercive Acts to bring them into line. Within twelve months this would precipitate the eight bloody years of the American War of Independence and a dramatic change in the history of the world.

Things seemed better at home. Back in the early 1700s, the bulk of the population had lived as their forefathers did, accepting their lot within the sharp division of rich and poor. When discontent festered, the populace expressed its feelings by rioting. Riots over such diverse matters as food, silk weaving or the introduction of road tolls had been tolerated as necessary aspects of life. Thankfully, matters were now improving. There had been a huge increase in the population. The emergence of business and professional enterprise was leading to the creation of a new middle class, though this remained disparate in wealth and activity. Cities were cleaner and there was much rebuilding. Sewers and water mains had been laid. There was pride in the new architecture. The Royal Crescent in Bath was ready for occupation in 1774, and Capability Brown completed his finest landscape garden at Blenheim Palace. Invention and inspiration flourished. Richard Arkwright found premises for the commercial production of his Spinning Jenny. James Watt perfected a reliable version of Newcomen's steam engine. Chlorine was discovered by the Swede, Karl Scheele, and Joseph Priestley reported finding oxygen. John Hunter began to give lectures to students on the principles of surgery. Mesmer first used hypnosis. Captain James Cook was continuing his explorations on the far side of the world. In London, rules were revised for a new and mysterious sporting recreation – the game of cricket. The author and poet Robert Southey was born in the same year. Among Southey's works would be his biography 'The Life of the Rev Andrew Bell'. This book was to contain details of the Rev Bell's encounter with a farmer who had a remarkable story to tell. The farmer's name was Benjamin Jesty.

Benjamin Jesty was born in 1736 at the village of Yetminster, near Sherborne, in the county of Dorset. The original family name was Justy, and why it was changed is a mystery. Benjamin's grandfather was named John Justy. He lived at Leigh, near Yetminster, and was a fairly wealthy man. John's son, Robert Justy, was a butcher who had at least four sons. One was christened Benjamin at Yetminster on the 19th August 1736, and the boy was probably educated in the village school which had been endowed by Robert Boyle FRS. The date of the change of surname is unknown. Benjamin signed himself as Jesty when he was a witness to a marriage in 1763, and at his own wedding in 1770. The family must have approved. The rest of them gradually adopted the new surname and the name Justy disappeared.

Benjamin and his growing family lived at Upbury, a large stone farmhouse of medieval origin still to be found next to St Andrew's Church in Yetminster. Upbury is thought to be the oldest house in the village and is set well back from Church Street, next to the sexton's cottage. There is a large cobbled yard in front, with a number of barns and buildings bordering the property. Upbury was the capital messuage of one of the four Yetminster manors, probably built by the prebends of Salisbury Cathedral as country retreats. The two blocked and trefoiled windows at the front of the house are immediately obvious. These may date from the 15th century but are not in their original positions. The dwelling has been subjected to a series of reconstructions at various times in its history, but the original medieval house consisted of a central open hall, accessed by opposing doors and bounded by two-storied rooms at each end. I once had the good fortune to be taken on a brief tour of the ground floor of Upbury. We entered through a stone doorway into an entrance hall, leading to a lateral passage which ran the length of the building at the rear. Stairs at one end led to the upper storey.

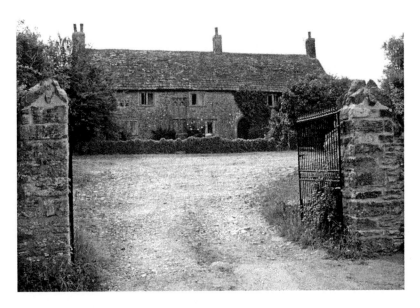

Upbury Farmhouse in Yetminster. Benjamin Jesty was living here in 1774

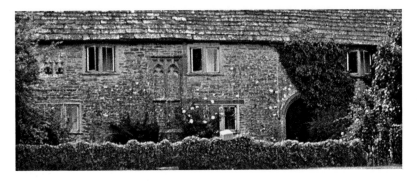

Front elevation of Upbury showing some of the detail described in the text.

The overwhelming impression was that of age. The heavy oak doors must certainly have been there in Jesty's day. The large fireplaces had been modernised but it was easy to imagine the farmer and his family gathered round the hearth on a cold winter evening. Period furnishings complemented the atmosphere perfectly. The central position of the property in Church Street is easily explained. In the Georgian era it was usual for a farmhouse to be situated among the other village buildings, with the associated fields scattered throughout the neighbouring countryside. Upbury is still a working farm today. Cattle were being driven from the yard on their way out to pasture at the time of my visit.

Jesty reached the age of 38 in 1774 and had been married for four years to his wife Elizabeth (née Notley). They had two sons at this time - Robert (3 yrs) and Benjamin (2 yrs) - and their baby daughter Betty, who had been born the year before. These were revolutionary days in the approach to farming. The enclosure system had led to new crops such as potatoes being grown on a commercial scale. Townshend introduced the concept of crop rotation. Seed quality had improved, and Jethro Tull had invented the seed drill. Cattle were now bred for the production of meat and leather, rather than just for dairy products. This new enterprise was assisted by another development - the growing of crops specifically intended for the provision of fodder during the winter months. Farmers thrived on innovation and many emerged as the *nouveau riche* of the day.

Jesty was an intelligent man and, like other professionals, had responsibilities to the local parish. He was a member of the Yetminster Vestry and his duties included making provision for the healthcare of the local poor. Smallpox was a constant threat as the 'Speckled Monster' ebbed and flowed throughout the 1700s. The number of deaths from smallpox each year in Europe during this period has been estimated to be at least 400,000. Repeated outbreaks affected populations both in cities and in the rural areas. The only means of reducing the impact of epidemic infection at that time was the perilous process of inoculation. Faced with an outbreak of smallpox that had begun at the end of 1771 the Yetminster Vestry decided that something should be done despite the inherent hazards. An extract from their minutes of the 9th February 1772 proclaims:

'…on Mature Consideration respecting the present danger the Poor of the said Parish are in who have not had the smallpox, and of the probability of the said Distemper spreading in the Parish in its natural course and for the purpose of preserving the lives of such as choose to receive our advice and will put themselves under the care and Direction of some Surgeon of Eminence in the practice of Innoculation, do hereby consent and agree that such of the Parish as think fit shall be Innoculated at the expense of our said Parish'.

Smallpox was present in Jesty's locality again during the latter half of 1774. Country tales of cattle workers somehow becoming resistant to smallpox after acquiring cowpox were commonplace amongst the farming communities. Whilst many people carried facial scars as witness to their survival from smallpox infection, dairymaids were noted for their unblemished complexions – hence the traditional air;

> 'Where are you going to my pretty maid?
> I'm going a-milking, Sir, she said,
> What is your fortune, my pretty maid?
> My face is my fortune, Sir, she said'.

Cowpox only exists in Europe and those countries which once formed the Soviet Union. The virus is a member of the Poxvirus family. It has the same size and shape as the smallpox virus but differs in the make-up of its genome and constituent parts. The natural reservoir of cowpox is in wild rodents, particularly woodmice and bank voles. Cowpox can infect a wide range of mammals including cows, cats, some zoo animals, and also humans. Nowadays, humans are more likely to acquire cowpox from cats. Feline infection tends to peak in the autumn when small rodents are more active, though the number of human cases of cowpox recorded in the UK rarely exceeds 2 or 3 per annum at the present time. Bovine cowpox is now extremely rare. In the eighteenth century it was more widespread, probably because of the large workforce involved in agriculture, their close association with cattle, and a lack of understanding of the biology of the disease. The symptoms manifest in the cow as lesions on the udder or teats, and humans contract the disease by having contact with an infected beast during milking or animal husbandry. The disease in humans is mild, and usually seen as a single pustular lesion which arises after 9 - 10 days incubation at the site of introduction of virus into the skin – most commonly on the thumb or forefinger. This may be accompanied by a slight fever, with myalgia (muscle pain) in occasional cases.

Jesty had acquired cowpox whilst working with cattle in his youth. His notion of cowpox preventing smallpox was strengthened through discussion with two of his dairymaids, Anne Notley and Mary Reade. Both had been infected with cowpox as a result of milking cows. Neither of them had contracted smallpox thereafter, even when nursing relatives with the disease. Jesty was convinced that the folklore was true. Confident that he had thought of a safe way to protect his family, Jesty took his wife and two sons to a farm where he knew some cows had the marks of cowpox on their udders. These cattle were in the ownership of a farmer named Elford and were grazing near the neighbouring village of '*Chittenhall*' – the Dorset dialect pronunciation of Chetnole. On reaching the herd, Jesty searched their teats for signs of cowpox. He took material from a lesion onto the tip of a stocking needle and transferred this to his wife's arm, inserting it into her skin immediately below the elbow. He then repeated this for Robert and Benjamin, making punctures just above the elbow in each case. Jesty's venture came to light when a problem arose. Signs of inflammation appeared at the site of Elizabeth's vaccination. Medical assistance was summoned immediately from nearby Cerne – both Mr Henry Meech and Dr Trowbridge are mentioned in the records. Jesty told them about his cowpox experiment. Trowbridge replied, 'You have done a bold thing, but I will get you through if I can', and treated Elizabeth's condition as a fever. She recovered completely.

Word of the deed spread throughout Dorset and became well known in the medical, farming and ecclesiastical communities. Jesty became the object of scorn and derision. He suffered verbal and physical abuse for some time afterwards when he attended markets. Many regarded him as an inhuman brute. The very idea of transferring matter from a mere beast into the body of a human was contrary to everything they had been taught from the pulpit about the sanctity of *Homo sapiens*, created in

God's own image. Darwin's Theory of Evolution was a hundred years in the future and country people were very suspicious of anything which seemed alien to their traditional beliefs. The last execution for witchcraft had taken place only 62 years before. Jesty steadfastly continued with his parish duties, ignoring the unwelcome attention. The trio of vaccinees remained free of smallpox for the rest of their lives, though often exposed to epidemics of the disease. The two sons were inoculated with smallpox by Dr Trowbridge in 1789. Robert, then aged 18 years, and Benjamin, 17 years, were unaffected – showing that they had developed immunity to the virus. It is reasonable to assume that their proven immunity had been stimulated by the cowpox vaccinations given to them by their father, but, like Jenner's work, this cannot be confirmed scientifically in retrospect. The 1802 investigation into the farmer's actions is described in Chapter 5.

Jesty's family retained a sense of pride in his bold deed, despite the misguided reactions of the local folk. On the 27th June 1832, the surgeon and geologist, Gideon Mantell, was undertaking a coach journey from Bristol to Lyme Regis. He describes the trip in great detail in his *Journal*. The coach stopped at the village of Clutton, which lies 9 miles south of Bristol. Mantell continues his narrative as follows:

'A person here took his seat by the side of me who informed me that his name was Jesty, that his father practised vaccination as early as Jenner, and he himself was in fact the first (male) person ever vaccinated intentionally: that his father was sent for to London by some opponents of Dr Jenner and that he also remained in town a considerable time; but ultimately the affair was dropped, when it was found Parliament would not grant any money to any claimant but Jenner. Mr Jesty was a shrewd and intelligent farmer and amused us much with his droll remarks'.
from The Journal of Gideon Mantell, Ed. 1940 E C Curwen, by permission of Oxford University Press

Mantell had been privileged to hear a first hand account of the vaccination event from Benjamin's eldest son, Robert Jesty, who was then aged 61. The surgeon must have considered the anecdote significant enough to make room for it in his book. Like him, I was intrigued and felt that Marjorie Wallace's story of Jesty warranted further investigation. I began to make regular visits to the beautiful county of Dorset, where I had the lasting pleasure of getting to know Bill, Vera, and other members of the present Jesty family. I embarked upon a journey of exploration through repositories of archives and reference libraries in Dorset and London. The resourcefulness of the inventive Benjamin Jesty had kindled my admiration, and I wanted to dig a little deeper.

Before proceeding further, it might be helpful to clarify the differences between two items of terminology used frequently in these chapters in an historical context :

Inoculation – the deliberate infection of a person with live **smallpox** virus that had been collected from the skin lesions of a patient suffering from the mild form of the disease - Lady Mary's 'best sort of smallpox'! Infection was achieved by seeding superficial incisions made in the recipient's skin with a lancet. Either fresh smallpox lymph or powder prepared from dried scabs was used. Some practitioners preserved material on short lengths of thread and these could be inserted into incisions.

Vaccination – the deliberate transfer of **cowpox** virus to a human, by insertion into the skin using one of a number of types of needle, or lancet. The virus was contained in lymph collected from a lesion on the udder or teat of a cow that displayed typical signs of cowpox. As we shall see later, another option was to obtain lymph from human cases of cowpox. Material for vaccination could also be preserved in a dried state by impregnating threads with cowpox lymph. These were applied to a person's skin as mentioned above. Vaccination is sometimes confusingly referred to as 'inoculation for the cow pox' in old books and documents.

Keen to establish the exact location of Jesty's historic event, I sought advice from the Hundred of Yetminster Local History Society. Mrs Nina Hayward replied, sending me a list of field names that had been associated with the local Elford family in the eighteenth century. I searched the Yetminster Court records at the Dorset Archives Service and confirmed that four of the listed field names were associated with the farmer, William Elford, at the time of Jesty's vaccinations. The tradition of naming fields goes back at least to medieval times, and names are sometimes derived from Latin or Old English. It was no surprise to find field names linked with the Elfords entered on a Tithe Map of Chetnole drawn seventy years later. I noted that some adjoining fields shown on this map shared the same names. Most of the field boundaries can still be traced on the current Ordnance Survey Explorer Map of the area. These pastures are in close proximity to a property known as Foys in Chetnole village, which lies 3.7 km (2.3 miles) from the home of Benjamin Jesty. William Elford Snr. lived at Chetnole farm with his wife, Mary. They produced four sons, one being named John Foy Elford. Mary is also mentioned in connection with Foys in the Deeds of the Elford family, though this cannot be the existing building.

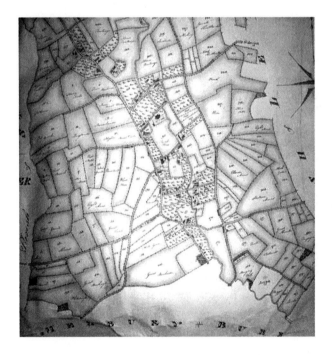

Field boundaries on a Tithe Map of Chetnole village in Dorset
Reproduced from the Chetnole Tithe Map 1840 – 41
held at the Dorset History Centre (reference T/CHN)

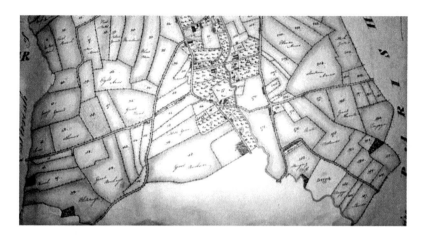

Detail of fields on Chetnole Tithe Map (T/CHN) – compare with the map below.

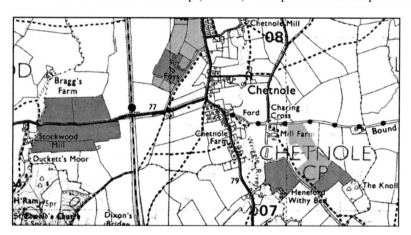

Fields in the same area seen on an extract from a modern Ordnance Survey Map.
Dark grey fill = fields recorded in Deeds of the Elford family up to 1774.
Light grey fill = fields also mentioned in a later Sale of a William Elford's Estate.

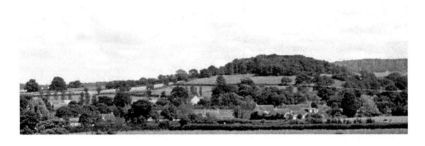

View of fields below The Knoll at the South-East of Chetnole village that were farmed by William Elford in 1774. These are indicated on the lower right of extracts from the Tithe and Ordnance Survey maps seen on the previous page.

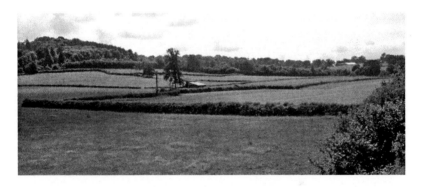

View of fields below Melbury Bubb at the South-West of Chetnole village that were farmed by William Elford in 1774. These are indicated at the lower left of extracts from the Tithe and Ordnance Survey maps seen on the previous page.

The fields shown in the photographs are all found in close proximity to the River Wriggle and lie at a distance of 3.7 km (2.3 miles) from Upbury farmhouse in Yetminster village. Benjamin Jesty came here in 1774 with his wife and two sons to vaccinate them with cowpox taken from the teats of infected cows that were owned by William Elford.

Primed with this information, I went to Chetnole to explore the location of the world's first vaccination. Elford's fields are set between the wooded slopes of Melbury Bubb and The Knoll, bisected by the River Wriggle. These fields are clustered at OS Grid References 594074, 600078 and 607072. This landscape has changed little since Jesty's day. The Yeovil/Dorchester railway track is the obvious exception. My visit proved more than a mere pilgrimage of curiosity. Whilst taking time to absorb the scenery, I realised I could barely see the tower of St Andrew's Church in distant Yetminster away to the north. The material reality of the map measurement brought a new perspective to the situation. The distance from Upbury to Elford's fields bears witness to the extent of Jesty's foresight and planning. What happened here was no fleeting daydream of some country bumpkin; it required inspiration and a firm resolve.

I felt Jesty's enterprise merited closer scrutiny in the light of the new information. This shrewd farmer believed that contracting cowpox disease would somehow protect an individual against smallpox. He had formed the idea that this would also happen if someone was deliberately 'given' cowpox. Though this might seem obvious to us now, it represents extraordinary perception for someone who was living in the eighteenth century, especially a rural layman with no medical education. Jesty decided he could achieve his aims by replacing smallpox material with that of cowpox as an effective and safer form of inoculation. The project must have been discussed with his immediate family. Baby Betty was not to be included. She was considered to be too young and remained at Upbury, probably in the care of the dairymaid Anne Notley. The records suggest that Anne was Jesty's wife's cousin, and she was living with the family at Upbury in 1774. Jesty had to access the cowpox in Elford's herd. My investigations show this could only be achieved by the family covering a minimum total distance of 7.4 km (4.6 miles) for the round trip. Any father or mother will appreciate the practical problems of transporting children - a two-year-old and a three-year-old - over this distance. The Rev Andrew Bell's account, based on a conversation with Jesty himself, states that 'Mr Jesty carried his family'. This suggests that the parents may have walked to Chetnole with the children in their arms, but even if some form of conveyance had been used, this would have required the harnessing of a horse to a cart or trap. Either situation indicates considered intent rather than whimsical fancy.

Jesty equipped himself with a stocking needle before setting out. This type of needle was widely used for the hand knitting of hose in the area around Sturminster Newton and other parts of Dorset. Here, the local craft remained a thriving cottage industry, in contrast to machine knitting, which had been introduced in some Midland counties. Jesty's wife came from nearby Longburton. She would have learnt the traditional skills in her youth and most certainly knitted knee length stockings for her husband with such needles. The slender point would have pierced skin easily. In Thomas Hardy's *The Return of the Native,* Susan Nunsuch pricks the arm of Eustacia Vye with 'a long stocking needle'. Susan's intention was to draw blood! In Book the Third, chapter 3 of the novel, we are given a brief description of the healing wound:

'Eustacia slowly drew up her sleeve and disclosed her round white arm. A bright red spot appeared on its surface, like a ruby on Parian marble'.

Clym is mentioned as 'looking at the scarlet little puncture'.

A review of former vaccination instruments and techniques was published by Baxby in 2002. He identified eleven different methods and listed them in chronological order. Puncture of the epidermis could be achieved by stabbing the skin with a round needle. This was an early alternative to the linear cut or scratch obtained with a lancet. The needle was used by holding it at right angles to the skin surface, Vaccination by puncture with a steel needle was an option in the US Army into the 20th Century. Spring powered needles were marketed up till 1935. They could be adjusted for depth of penetration.

It is important to consider the magnitude of Jesty's endeavour, when set against the proclivities of society at the time. Today, medicine is often described as an art as well as a science, but in the eighteenth century the scientific basis of this discipline was in its infancy. There was much quackery. The only British medical schools were in London and Edinburgh, so there were few doctors who had received a formal education and there was no unifying standard. The majority received their training through several years of apprenticeship with an apothecary and they became healers who perpetuated the old traditions. Transported back in time, we would find it difficult to distinguish the quacks from some of the legitimate practitioners. Most qualified doctors had a basic knowledge of anatomy but not of how the various parts of the body actually worked. Healers relied greatly upon the traditions of folk medicine. Treatment often involved the application of a succession of curatives until one produced a positive response.

It was at this time that hospitals began to be founded specifically for the care of those with illness, and when medical personnel began to take the responsibility for governing them. These establishments differed from the hospices that had been provided by religious orders for centuries as refuges for the chronically sick. The new hospitals were staffed by a complement of physicians, surgeons and apothecaries. Nurses were akin to household servants. Women also acted as midwives, but the 'learned' men of medicine took great care to maintain their profession as a male preserve, with an aura of mystique. This is one reason why the physicians always wrote in Latin.

Bacteria and viruses were unknown, although Anthony Van Leeuwenhoek had reported to the Royal Society on the 17th September 1683 that he had seen 'very little animalcules a-swimming' when he inspected white matter from the plaque of his teeth under his primitive microscope. A little earlier, the Jesuit, Athanasius Kirchner, had proposed that the 'beasties' he saw with his early microscope might be the cause of disease but he was discredited by his colleagues because their less proficient instruments failed to detect the organisms. The science of microbiology did not really emerge until the late 19th century. Microbes, disinfectants and antibiotics were not even the figments of someone's imagination in Jesty's era.

The 1700s were truly an Age of Enlightenment and the medical profession promised an exclusive, not to say lucrative, career. Treatment was often a haphazard, painful or ineffective experience for the patient. News of a humble farmer coming forward with a new idea for protecting against 'a distemper' would have been dismissed as preposterous by the professionals, and viewed with considerable animosity by the general public. The outcome of Jesty's '*bold thing*' resulted in him being reviled by the local population. Learning that of one of their number had introduced matter from a beast of the field into the body of a human being would have evoked strong moral and religious taboos. Bell records that the prejudice against Jesty was carried to such a height that a surgeon (presumably Trowbridge) 'almost lost his practice' from following up the results of the experiment. In addition to the personal anguish he must have felt over Elizabeth's post-vaccination reaction, Jesty paid a high price for his ingeniousness. Undaunted, he valiantly continued his farming business and attended to his parish duties in the face of a constant atmosphere of abhorrence and suspicion. He did nothing to publicise the merits of his experiment and refrained from conducting further vaccinations whilst living in Yetminster. This is wholly understandable. Jesty moved out of the area in later years, as we shall see in the next chapter. Through his relocation came an encounter which led to a recognition of sorts, and the first move towards securing his place in the history of medicine.

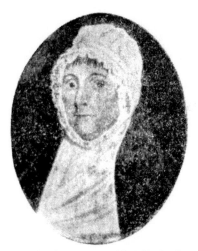

Benjamin Jesty's wife Elizabeth
the first person known to be vaccinated.

Chapter 5

Pastures New

A mile to the west of Yetminster lies the hamlet of Ryme Intrinseca (*der., within the estate of Ryme*). A new rector arrived in the parish in 1793. His name was the Rev Morgan Jones, a clergyman who also held a living at Worth Matravers, near Swanage. His dual appointment is recorded on a tablet in Ryme church. Jones travelled regularly between the two parishes, funding the rebuilding of the parsonage at Ryme from his own pocket. This commuting minister would have often met Benjamin Jesty in the course of his duties, and it seems that during one of their conversations he told Jesty of a vacant tenancy of a farm in the Isle of Purbeck. The farm was at Downshay Manor, situated close to Harman's Cross, a short distance from Swanage. Jesty moved there with his family around 1796/97 – the record is incomplete. One can only speculate at the reason for the relocation. The farm was larger, the accommodation more spacious, and he would be able to escape from the undeserved hostility that had been harboured in the minds of some Yetminster folk for over twenty years. Another factor could have been a change in his tenancy of Upbury. Thomas Lydiat had become Lord of the Manor of Yetminster Prima in 1796. Perhaps Jesty was unhappy with something associated with his new landlord. Maybe the lease had run its course. Certainly he left abruptly, without leaving some fences and gates in good order as custom demanded, and was required to make reparation after his departure. The next tenant of Upbury, one Samuel Eastment, constantly made excuses that he was unable to pay his rent for one reason or another, and Lydiat complains of not receiving his dues.

Downshay Manor is a beautiful old house, built of stone from the local quarries. It was constructed by the Dolling family in 1642 and is not open to the public. The name Dolling (also featured in a later chapter of the Jesty story) is commemorated by initials on the rainwater heads and stone window frames.

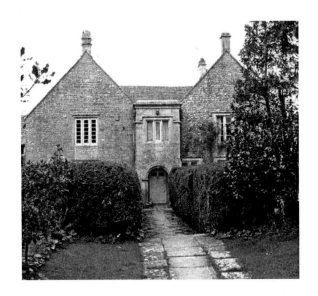

Downshay Manor (Dunshay) east elevation. The north wing was rebuilt in 1906. Benjamin Jesty lived here from 1796/97 until his death in 1816.

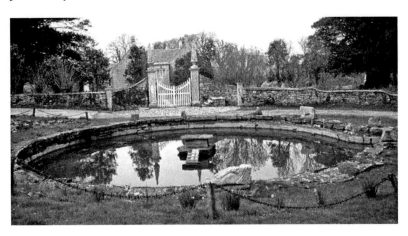

The pond fronting the gates of Downshay Manor, with the house just visible behind the stone pillars. Note the mounting block which would have been used by Jesty when he set out for London on horseback in 1805.

The house is secreted away in a small valley where time seems to have stood still. The driveway descends through trees and banks of wild flowers to widen out into a cobbled courtyard with a central pond. The gates of Downshay are hung from two distinctive stone posts capped with tall pyramidal obelisks. A mounting block is set close to one of these posts and has an old millstone as its platform. The house is roughly square on plan but has been subject to alteration over the centuries. Two gables flank a central porch on the east front. The north wing was in ruins in Jesty's time but was rebuilt in 1906. At the time of my visit, Downshay was owned by the late Miss Mary Spencer-Watson, a distinguished sculptress, who inherited the property from her father. I was privileged to be able to meet her during 2004. I found Miss Spencer-Watson to be an industrious nonagenarian who was still working and exhibiting. She had revived the ancient name of Dunshay for the manor house, which retains some original features including seventeenth century panelling and a fireplace. Miss Spencer-Watson died in March 2006.

Benjamin and Elizabeth were the proud parents of seven children by the time of the move. Robert, Benjamin and Betty had been joined by Thomas, Sarah, George and Harriet. Having settled the family into their new home, Jesty resumed his farming activities. Everyone living on the south coast must have been acutely aware of the increasing threat from recent happenings in France. Shortly after the architects of the French Revolution had been put to the guillotine, Napoleon Bonaparte rose to prominence as a military leader. He arrived in Paris in 1797, appointed to command forces for an invasion of England. The Peace of Amiens in 1802 brought a brief respite, then hostilities were renewed between France and England within a year. Parliament replaced the Militia Act of 1757 with that of 1802 and set up Defence Lists such as the Levée en Masse. These provided for both conscription and voluntary service. Jesty is listed in the Volunteer Rangers. He had special responsibilities as an overseer driver and was to 'take charge of livestock'. Such men were needed to support active fighting units on English soil in the event of a French landing. Benjamin Jesty Jnr and his brother Thomas enlisted in the yeomanry cavalry. Thankfully, an invasion did not take place and their participation in active service was not required.

In the spring of 1803 Jesty met the Rev Andrew Bell. Dr Bell was a celebrated man of letters who had distinguished himself in India, where he set up a self-help scheme of primary education for orphan children. Continuing this mission on his return to England, he introduced his 'Madras System' at St Botolph's School in Aldgate. He was appointed to the livings of Swanage and Worth Matravers in 1801 as places where he might enjoy some years of restful vocation. However, the founder and promoter of Free Schools found that the insular position of Swanage meant that social conditions in the locality gave great cause for concern. Dr Bell did all he could to improve matters, including the setting up of a profitable straw-plait cottage industry for the residents. It was now twenty-nine years since Jesty had vaccinated his family. By this time, Dr Edward Jenner had published the all-important *Inquiry*, describing his own experiments in Gloucestershire. Vaccination with cowpox was being adopted by many medical practitioners as a safer replacement for 'The Inoculation', its risky predecessor. Dr Bell had become an enthusiastic vaccinator and was dismayed to find that the efficacy of vaccination was still doubted by those living in the Isle of Purbeck. He brought some vaccine material from Edinburgh and started a campaign to popularise it immediately. Bell personally vaccinated large numbers of children and adults in and around Swanage. It was inevitable that he would encounter Benjamin Jesty at some point.

The clergyman's account of his meeting with Jesty is set down in great detail by the author, Robert Southey, in his biography *The Life of the Rev Andrew Bell* and is the closest we are able to get to the first vaccinator's own version of events. The rector was obviously very impressed with the farmer and the story of his enterprise. Bell emphasises that the extraordinary deeds of 1774,

'may be thought not unworthy of a place in the history of the cow-pox. If it should have any influence with those parents who decline the offer made to them of having their children vaccinated, my object is attained; and let Mr Jesty have that share of credit'.

The Rev Bell was motivated to take the matter further and immediately entered into correspondence on Jesty's behalf as described in a later chapter. His support continued and on Sunday the 15th July 1806 Bell preached the same sermon twice in honour of the man,

'whose discovery of the efficacy of the cowpock against smallpox is so often forgotten by those who have heard of Dr Jenner'.

Little did he know that his words would ring true, not only during the early nineteenth century, but also for many years reaching up to the beginning of the present Millenium.

Soon after Bell's intercession, Benjamin Jesty received a letter dated 25th July 1805. It was an invitation to visit London. This came from the secretary of the Original Vaccine Pock Institution, Will Sancho. Jesty accepted the invitation and called upon his neighbour, the father of the Rev J.M.Colson, to borrow some saddle-bags for the transport of clean shirts. He was promptly advised that saddlebags would be considered '*extinctum genus*' in the City. Colson senior (whose surname is entered on Taylors 1765 map of Dorset for Afflington Farm, near Dunshay) supplied him with a portmanteau as a more suitable and convenient vehicle. Benjamin's family tried to persuade him that he should attire himself more fashionably as he was going to the capital but to no avail. He exclaimed that 'he did not see why he should dress better in London than in the country' and accordingly wore his usual clothing, which was rather old-fashioned. Jesty was accompanied by his eldest son, Robert (by then 28 years old). They duly arrived at the offices of the Institution, then situated close to Regent Street at 44 Broad Street, Golden Square.

The Vaccine Pock Institution had been founded on the 2nd December 1799 at Warwick Street, near Charing Cross. The organisation moved to 'a more commodious house' at 5 Golden Square in April 1801 then finally on to Broad Street. The address at the time of Jesty's visit is a little confusing, as there was no Broad Street in the square itself. However, in Georgian times it was fashionable for the residents of all the neighbouring streets to include Golden Square in their addresses. The building which housed the Vaccine Pock Institution may be seen in Woolnoth's engraving of Broad Street on the extreme right of the picture, where two ladies are walking past some railings bordering the rear edge of the pavement. Number 44 was on the corner of Broad Street and Poland Street, situated directly opposite the Broad Street water pump, also shown

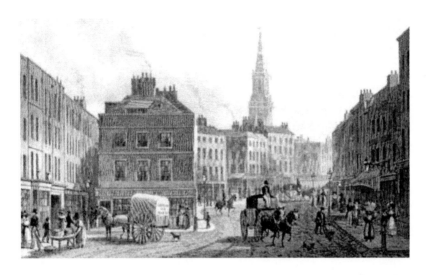

Broad Street, London, as it appeared in Georgian times. This engraving by Woolnoth shows where the Original Vaccine Pock Institution was sited in 1805 at the time of Jesty's visit – note the tall building at the extreme right of the picture.

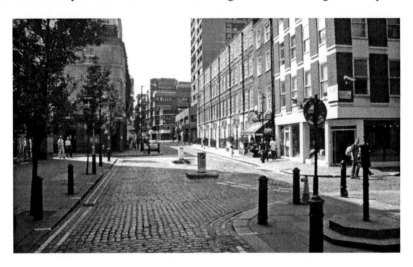

Broad Street, now renamed Broadwick Street, as it is today

in the engraving. This pump was to become the focus of an outbreak of cholera in 1854. The physician, John Snow, is credited with founding the science of epidemiology when he plotted the geographical distribution of cases on a map. He then deduced that the water from the pump was contaminated, and removed the handle from the pump to prevent further infections. Today, the street is named Broadwick Street. Number 44 was destroyed in the 1939-45 war, and is now a modern building, but an adjacent Georgian terrace remains and was dated 1723 by Pevsner.

The two Dorset men met with much attention from the members of the society, who were greatly amused by Benjamin's manners and appearance. Jesty was not enthusiastic about the metropolis, but admitted the one great comfort was that he could be shaved every day instead of wearing a beard from Saturday to Saturday. Normally he would only shave before attending the weekly market in Wareham. The physicians, surgeons and apothecaries of the Institution questioned Jesty about his vaccination 'experiment', listened to his reasoning, and received permission for Robert to be publicly inoculated with live smallpox in order to prove he was still protected against the disease. Jesty had developed a plausible hypothesis for vaccination with cowpox out of his conversations with the milkmaids at Upbury – an idea deduced from his own observations and the application of rural logic. This is made clear in the answers he gave when examined by the officials of the Institute in August 1805. Twelve of the Institute's examining officers were signatories to a statement commemorating the 'antivariolus efficacy' of Jesty's cowpox vaccinations. This was issued from their establishment at No. 44 Broad Street in London on the 6th September 1805 and published in the *Edinburgh Medical and Surgical Journal* soon after:

'Mr Benjamin Jesty, farmer of Downshay, in the Isle of Purbeck, having (agreeably to an invitation from the Medical Establishment of the Original Vaccine Pock Institution, Broad Street, Golden Square) visited London in August 1805 to communicate certain facts relating to the Cow Pock Institution, we think it a matter of justice to himself, and beneficial to the public, to attest that, among other facts, he has afforded decisive evidence of his having vaccinated his wife and two sons, Robert and

Benjamin, in the year 1774; who were thereby rendered unsusceptible of the small-pox, as appears from the exposure of all the three parties to that disorder frequently during the course of 31 years, and from the inoculation of the two sons for the small-pox fifteen years ago. That he was led to undertake this novel practice in 1774, to counteract the small-pox, at that time prevalent at Yetminster, where he then resided, from knowing the common opinion of the country, ever since he was a boy (now 60 years ago), that persons who had gone through the cow-pock naturally, *i.e.* by taking it from cows, were unsusceptible of the small-pox; by himself being incapable of taking the small-pox, having gone through the cow-pock many years before; from having personally known many individuals, who, after the cow-pock, could not have the small-pox excited; from believing that the cow-pock was an affection free from danger; and from his opinion that, by the cow-pock inoculation, he should avoid ingrafting various diseases of the human constitution, such as "the Evil, madnes, lues, and many bad humours," as he called them.

The remarkable vigorous health of Mr. Jesty, his wife and two sons, now 31 years subsequent to the cow-pock, and his own healthy appearance, at this time 70 years of age, afford a singularly strong proof of the harmlessness of that affection; but the public must, with particular interest, hear that, during the late visit to town, Mr Robert Jesty very willingly submitted publicly to inoculation for the small-pox in the most rigorous manner; and that Mr. Jesty also was subjected to the trial of inoculation for the cow-pock after the most efficacious mode, without either of them being infected. The circumstances on which Mr. Jesty purposely instituted the vaccine-pock inoculation in his own family, – viz. **without any precedent**, but merely from reasoning upon the nature of the affection among cows, and from knowing its effects in the casual way among men, his exemption from the prevailing popular prejudices, and his disregard of the clamorous reproaches of his neighbours, in our opinion, will entitle him to the respect of the public for his superior strength of mind. But, further, his conduct in again furnishing such decisive proofs of the permanent antivariolous efficacy of the cow-pock, on the present discontented state of mind in many families, by submitting to inoculation, justly claims at least the gratitude of the country. As a testimony of our personal regard, and to commemorate so extraordinary a fact, as that of preventing the small-pox by inoculating for the cow-pock 31 years ago, at our request, a three quarter length picture of Mr Jesty is painted by that excellent artist Mr Sharp, to be preserved at the Original Vaccine Pock Institution'.

Geo.Pearson, Law.Nihell, Thos. Nelson – Physicians
T.Keate, T. Forster – Consulting Surgeons
Joseph.Constantine.Carpue, J.Doratt – Surgeons
Fras.Rivers, Ev.A.Brande, Ph.De Bruge – Visiting Apothecaries
John Heaviside, Thomas Payne – Treasurers   William Sancho – Secretary

The statement is reproduced here as a direct transcription from the original publication, with the exception of the letter 's', which appears as 'f' in the document. The reader will see from the statement that Jesty saw an element of danger in transferring cowpox lymph from one person to another. The *'Evil'* (the King's Evil) was the term for scrofula, and *'Lues'* was syphilis. He was entirely correct in his opinion – Bazin gives an estimate of approximately 750 cases of syphilis occurring in 100 million arm-to-arm vaccinations, yet this approach was not prohibited until 1898. Jesty's reasoning would still be respected today. When the first Hepatitis B vaccine was introduced in 1981, many were wary of receiving it. The purified vaccine was declared safe, but it had been prepared from blood donated by those who had had the infection. There was always the possibility that these donors might have had other diseases as well – perhaps some unknown to medicine at the time, as was HIV. It is understandable that Jesty, a dairy farmer, preferred to take cowpox directly from the cow. His simple explanation is convincing:

'There is little risk in introducing into the human constitution matter from the cow as we already without danger eat the flesh and blood, drink the milk and cover ourselves with the skin of this innocuous animal'.

Not wholly 'innocuous' of course, for milk was always a potential source of tuberculosis at that time. The most likely hazard arising from transferring cowpox lymph directly from a cow's udder to human skin by incision would not have come from tuberculosis but from contaminating bacteria that might predispose to sepsis spreading from the site of vaccination. This was the most likely cause of Elizabeth's fever. Despite the inherent drawbacks, vaccination 'on the hoof' became popular in some countries such as France where a cowpox infected calf would be led into the room as a ready source of lymph. This eliminated the hazards of arm-to-arm transfer but the vaccination clinic cannot have presented a very edifying spectacle for those attending.

I would now like to present a comprehensive provenance of Jesty's portrait. This contains new information which has relevance to his status as an historical figure. The 'excellent artist' commissioned by the Vaccine Pock Institute was Michael W Sharp (op 1801-1840) of 22 Marlborough Street, London. Sharp was a notable painter of his day, whose works included the first Duke of Wellington. Jesty proved to be an impatient sitter, and only kept quiet when the artist's wife played to him upon the piano. The completed painting, which forms the colour frontispiece of this book, was first exhibited in Somerset House. The Institution also presented Jesty with a pair of gold mounted lancets, a testimonial scroll and the sum of fifteen guineas for his expenses.

The oil painting was then removed from Somerset House and hung at the Original Vaccine Pock Institute as first intended. At some time when the painting was at the Institute, a monochrome engraving of the portrait was made in mezzotint by William Say and multiple copies were taken. Say (op c1800-1833) lived in London. He specialised in portraits, having already made one of Jenner from the painting of him by Northcote, and was probably the leading British engraver at the time. His works included George III and George IV and he had been appointed engraver to the Duke of Gloucester in 1807. An inscription was set at the foot of the Jesty engraving which reads as follows:

'To the President, Vice Presidents, Treasurers, Trustees and Medical Officers of the Original Vaccine Institution. This print of Mr Benjamin Jesty, from a picture in the possession of the Institution, is respectfully inscribed by their devoted servant, William Say. Mr Benjamin Jesty,

Farmer of Downshay, Isle of Purbeck *aet.* 70, who inoculated his Wife and Two Sons for the Vaccine Pock in 1774, from his cows, at that time disorder'd by the Cow Pock, and who subsequently from the most rigorous Trials have been found unsusceptible of the Smallpox. Having rationally set the example of Vaccine Inoculation from his own knowledge of the Fact of Unsusceptibility of the Smallpox after casual Cow Pock in his own Person and in that of others, and from knowing the harmlessness of the Complaint. To commemorate the Author of these historical truths the vaccine Institution have procured this Portrait'.

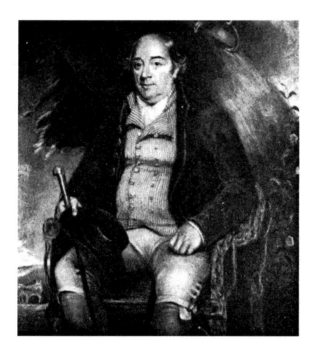

William Say's mezzotint engraving of Benjamin Jesty.
This interpretation of Jesty's character should be compared with the original oil portrait from which the engraving was prepared - see the colour frontispiece.

Signatories to this inscription were the same as those penned to the Vaccine Pock Institution's statement above. Edward Jenner complains about this in a letter to Dr Moore of the National Vaccine Institute:

'...his (Dr Pearson's) treatment of me before the committee of the House of Commons, the portrait of the farmer from the Isle of Purbeck with the farmer's claim to reward as the discoverer at the foot of it, with a thousand minor tricks'.

The Institution's fêting of Jesty is usually assumed to be a slight against the short lived Royal Jennerian Society. However, if the officers were merely seeking to make effective political capital against Jenner, they were too late. By the time of Jesty's visit to London, the Commons had already voted Jenner his first award and he was heavily involved in promoting and defending vaccination. Both the painter and engraver of Jesty's portrait were artists of high quality and would have charged accordingly for their services. Information regarding the impressive dimensions of the painting has never been published before. Still within what the owner presumes to be the original frame, the visible canvas measures 140 cms by 110 cms (55 inches by 43.25 inches). There is nothing written on the reverse of the canvas. An oil painting of this size by a noted London artist of the day would not have been a cheap option. This is also true of the commission for the preparation of an engraving by Say. It follows that the Institution was genuinely motivated, and prepared to go to considerable expense, in order to endow Benjamin Jesty with some form of official recognition as the first vaccinator. They sought to back their opinions with a lasting memorial of significant quality and size.

One of the engravings, or its photograph, was spotted on the 31st May 1862 by a surgeon, Mr Alfred Haviland, in the Rose and Crown Inn at Nether Stowey in Somerset. He describes the subject as 'a good specimen of the fine old English yeoman, dressed in knee breeches, extensive double-breasted waistcoat, and no small amount of broadcloth. He was represented sitting in an easy chair, under the shelter of some wide-spreading tree, with his stick and broad-brimmed hat in his left (*sic.*) hand; his ample frame surmounted by a remarkably good head, with a countenance which at once be-tokened firmness and superior intelligence'. It is not known if any of the original engravings survive. Those once seen in the vestry of the church at Worth Matravers in 1899, and the inn at Nether Stowey, have since disappeared.

After the closure of the Vaccine Pock Institute in 1807, the oil portrait was acquired by the Director, Dr George Pearson, and it was set up in his home. Coley has suggested that Pearson was the greatest chemist in England at this time. There is no doubt that he became a great rival to Jenner, and was very bitter about receiving insufficient recognition for his work in the early years of vaccination. One reason for this was the adverse publicity generated during an incident when some of his vaccine stocks were contaminated with smallpox material whilst in use.

The provenance of Jesty's oil portrait is complicated, but I have tried to compile a full account of its history. This proved to be a long and difficult task which required considerable resilience. The portrait was thought to be lost and nobody knew for certain if it still existed. I located it in October 2004 after a protracted search. Finding the painting was only made possible by the assistance I received from by a number of the people who are listed in the Acknowledgements. I am grateful to all of them for their kind co-operation, and their willingness to allow me to make the full story public.

Dr Pearson died in 1828 and the portrait was inherited by his son-in-law who gave it to Robert Jesty. Robert and his wife Edith lived at Wraxall House near Maiden Newton in Dorset. Their family of four children consisted of three sons and a daughter. The first son Edward died after one year, their second, Charles, remained a bachelor all his life, and the third son also named Edward, died when his was only ten. Edith, their daughter, married a man named Francis Pope on 23rd May 1844.

The portrait now passed out of ownership of the Jesty family. When Robert Jesty died in 1839 the portrait could not be given to the other recipient of Jesty's vaccination, his second son Benjamin, because he had died the year before. Edith (Robert's widow) gave it to her daughter, Edith, who had been married to Francis Pope for five years at that time. This is mentioned in a letter from London dated 18th June 1867 written by a Mr Say, who may well have been a descendant of the engraver. Francis and Edith Pope lived at Chilbridge Farm on the Kingston Lacy Estate near Wimborne Minster. Francis is listed in the 1861 Census as a farmer at Chilbridge, and also again in Kelly's Directory for Dorset in 1865. The 1861 records list six children. Two of their sons, one who was named William Percival Pope, were to emigrate to Cape Colony in South Africa in April 1878.

Francis Pope inherited another estate at Chilfrome on the death of his father, Ezekiel, in 1858. When Francis died in 1869 the estate passed to his eldest son, Frank Ezekiel Pope, who became the new owner of the portrait. He married his first cousin, Fanny Pope of Great Toller (Toller Porcorum) on the 9th January 1877. They continued to live at Chilfrome Manor House near Maiden Newton, a short distance from Toller. Frank is listed in Kelly's Directory at Chilfrome from 1875 onwards and is also entered as being there in the 1881 Census. It was confirmed that Benjamin's painting was in the possession of Frank Pope by Dr Edgar.M.Crookshank, who 'had the opportunity of seeing the portrait' during a visit to Chilfrome in 1888. Crookshank also acquired an engraving of the portrait, and a facsimile is reproduced as a frontispiece in his book *The History and Pathology of Vaccination* which was published in 1889.

Frank and Fanny died in 1919 and 1920 respectively. Their only child, Edward, had been killed in a tragic riding accident on his fourth birthday. As there was no direct heir, one of Edward's South African male cousins – Francis, a son of William Percival Pope - was appointed. Francis William Pope and his brother Tommy had been fighting in Europe with the South African Division during the First World War. Francis had taken the trouble to visit his aunt and uncle at Chilfrome whilst on leave from the Front, and was handsomely rewarded with his inheritance of their estate! When the war ended he returned to the family farm in the Eastern Cape Province of South Africa, then owned by Charles Frederick Pope. In 1934, Francis came to England and collected the family silver and pictures. He found the portrait of Benjamin Jesty in a barn. It was badly torn, so he had it restored in London and arranged for it to be transported to South Africa. The Chilfrome estate was sold in 1942 and the portrait became part of the Pope family home, being inherited by

Francis Stanley Pope in 1946. When Francis Stanley died in 1999 the painting was left to Charles Pope of Molteno, in the Eastern Cape.

I received colour photographs of the portrait from Charles in November 2004, and so became the first person outside the family to view the painting since Crookshank. A comparison of Say's image of Jesty in the engraving, copied from the original created in oils by Sharp, reveals some interesting differences. It is my opinion that Sharp's handling of the oil medium conveys a far more informative description of the subject. This is to be expected, as Sharp had Jesty sitting in front of him, whereas Say was reproducing a reversed copy of the painting on a copper plate as he engraved his mezzotint. Sharp gives us a competent image of a 68-year-old farmer who has been treated kindly by the passage of time. Weathered during long periods in the open air, Jesty's face bears a tanned complexion, with the exception of his balding forehead which has been paled by the wearing of a hat which he holds in his right hand. The pose is dignified and the portly sitter exudes an air of sturdiness and reliability. I feel that Jesty comes across as a no-nonsense character of determination and self-confidence, and this is not so apparent in the engraving.

I am delighted to report that Benjamin's oil portrait returned to England in June 2006, after it was purchased from Charles Pope by the Wellcome Library for the History of Medicine at Euston Road in London. This fitting memorial to a notable and perceptive layman will be seen once again in the city of its creation after an interval of 201 years.

Benjamin Jesty died on the 16th April 1816, seven years before Jenner. He lies next to his wife in the churchyard of St Nicholas of Myra in Worth Matravers, not far from Swanage in East Dorset. The inscription on his tombstone gives a posthumous publication of his vaccinations and reads:

'(Sacred) To the Memory of Benj.m Jesty, (of Downshay) who departed this Life, April 16th 1816 aged 79 years. He was born at Yetminster in this County, and was an upright honest Man: particularly noted for having been the first Person (known) that introduced the Cowpox by Inoculation, and who from his great strength of mind made the Experiment from the (Cow) on his Wife and two Sons in the Year 1774'

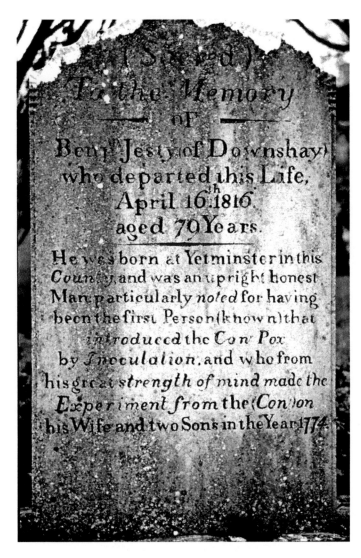

(Sacred)
To the Memory
— of —
Benj Jesty of Downshay,
who departed this Life,
April 16 1816.
aged 70 Years.

He was born at Yetminster in this
County, and was an upright honest
Man particularly noted for having
been the first Person (known) that
introduced the Cow Pox
by Inoculation, and who from
his great strength of mind made the
Experiment from the (Cow) on
his Wife and two Sons in the Year 1774

The epitaph on the tombstone of Benjamin Jesty.
He lies next to his wife, immediately behind the church of St Nicholas of Myra
at Worth Matravers near Swanage, in the Purbeck area of Dorset, England.

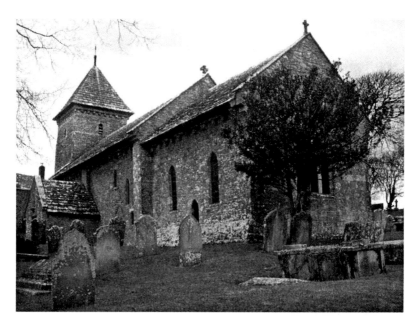

The church of St Nicholas of Myra at Worth Matravers. Jesty's grave is found by searching the area at the rear of the church seen in the far right of the photograph.

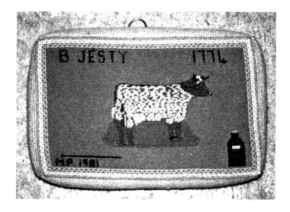

An unusual memorial to Benjamin Jesty found between the pews in St Nicholas Church. The embroidered kneeler made by Mrs Pike of Downshay Farm in 1981.

I had previously misinterpreted (see Lancet 2003) the words of an earlier account to believe that Jesty wrote his own epitaph. I now understand, from subsequent correspondence, that the inhabitants of Worth Matravers believe Elizabeth composed the entire inscription. Her inclusion of 'known' was an act of commendable integrity given the political infighting that was taking place amongst the medical fraternity at the time. However, when rumours of previous cowpox vaccinators in this country (or abroad) are subjected to careful scrutiny in the relevant literature, they are shown to be either smallpox inoculators, or individuals who proclaimed the protective effects of naturally acquired cowpox. I have made a special investigation of such claims, and in twenty-five years of research, I have found no reliable evidence to suggest that anyone predated Jesty in the practical use of vaccination.

James Moore, a staunch supporter of Jenner, published his *History and Practice of Vaccination* in 1817. He pays tribute to Jesty on page 147 of that book:

'This farmer cannot be denied the praise of having shown more medical acuteness than all the professional men around him. Yet the event of this inoculation from the cow was so far from leading to the practice of vaccination that it deterred both the farmer himself, and all the surgeons who had heard of it, from daring to repeat the experiment'.

Note: a plaque in the church of St Nicholas indicates that at least one further vaccination was performed by a Benjamin Jesty at a later date. This could have been undertaken by either the father or his son.

Moore's sentiments were echoed by Thomas McCrae, writing in the *Johns Hopkins Hospital Bulletin* in 1900:

'One feels that Jesty was in advance of his generation, and a man who saw probably better than he knew. He did his little to blaze out the path which has become a highway. That he could do but little to advance vaccination, his circumstances decided. To another was the honour of giving vaccination to the world'.

Chapter 6

The Enigmatic Doctor Jenner

I embarked upon this chapter with some trepidation because so much has been written about Dr Edward Jenner in the last two hundred years. His name has become inextricably linked throughout the world with the introduction of vaccination, and it would be over-ambitious in this small volume to present more than a synopsis of Jenner's great contribution to the advancement of medicine. The widespread populist acclaim has always been accompanied by a minority voice of dissension, and it was refreshing to hear searching questions on the iconic status of Jenner being asked by post-graduate historians at a meeting held as recently as 2005 within the hallowed portals of The Chantry itself. I would recommend the reader who wishes to explore his biography in some detail to examine the comprehensive and excellently researched literature of the other authors that I have listed in the Bibliography, though this represents only a fraction of the published works.

Jenner was born on the 26th May 1749 in Berkeley, Gloucestershire. The village is found bordering the upper reaches of that deep incision into the west coast of Britain which forms the Severn Estuary. The village is noted for its castle, where the barons of the West Country once put their signatures to the Magna Carta, and where the unfortunate Edward II was assassinated in 1327. Edward Jenner was the eighth child of the Rev Stephen Jenner, Vicar of Berkeley, and his wife Sarah. Only six of their children were to survive into adulthood. Edward was orphaned by the time he was five and went to live with his sisters, Mary, Sarah and Anne. In 1757 Mary married the new vicar, the Rev George Black. They sent eight-year-old Edward away in the same year to begin his education at Wotton-under-Edge Grammar School. This was a Free School for local boys whose parents could not afford to pay fees for the tuition of their children.

Soon after Edward arrived, the headmaster decided that Jenner, together with some of the other boys, should receive 'The Inoculation' as a safeguard against the smallpox which was present in the neighbourhood. The local 'surgeon', Mr Holbrow, used the long and arduous English version described in an earlier chapter. The process took six weeks. The young Jenner was reduced to a shadow of his former fitness by the preparation. He was then infected and is reported to have developed 'a terrible state of disease'. Fortunately, none of the boys died whilst forcibly confined in the school stables where they were housed for inoculation, but Edward retained the psychological effects of this trauma throughout his boyhood. He was placed in the care of a physician, Dr Capell, whilst at the school, and the event may have influenced his early departure.

Jenner left Wotton-under-Edge after only one year to become a boarding student in Cirencester. His new tutor, Dr Washbourne, taught him Latin, Greek and religious studies as a primer for entry to Oxford University. Edward made several friendships during this time and some of them lasted for the rest of his life. These included Caleb Parry who became a doctor based in the City of Bath. Edward was not a scholarly boy. He tolerated his lessons in the classics but was much more interested in natural history and geology. His room was full of collections of nests of dormice, various fossils and other items. He did not go to university and left Cirencester in 1761. It is not known who suggested that the adolescent Jenner should enter the medical profession. Probably, his interest in the natural world had been noticed, and the idea is thought to have originated from a close relative or family friend. Lack of a university education was not a problem. The first step on the medical ladder for many aspirants in those times was through apprenticeship to an apothecary.

Edward was accepted as an apprentice to the apothecary, Daniel Ludlow, when he was thirteen. Ludlow resided in the Cotswold village of Chipping Sodbury, and Jenner was to remain there for the next six years. He was made aware of the disease of cowpox towards the end of this time, 'about the year 1768'. A milkmaid told him how this could be contracted by persons milking infected cows, and said that they seemed to be protected afterwards from suffering the ravages of smallpox. Having completed his apprenticeship, Jenner could have now set up on his own as an apothecary. The title 'doctor' could only be used by practitioners who had taken a degree in 'physik' at Oxford or Cambridge, or by those who had purchased a degree from a Scottish university. There were further requirements for doctors who aspired to work in London.

Jenner decided to defer practice in favour of extending his medical studies, funding these in the same way as his apprenticeship, out of income derived from his inheritance. In 1770 he enrolled as a pupil of John Hunter at St George's Hospital in London. Hunter was the greatest surgeon of his time. Edward was among the first of his boarding pupils who were lodged at Hunter's home. He also attended classes run by Hunter's brother, William, at his school in Great William Street, and received instruction in midwifery by Denman and Osborne at St George's. These studies were complemented by attendance at lectures on chemistry, physics, and what is now known as pharmacology. Jenner was greatly influenced by Hunter's scientific approach to medicine. He taught that progress was associated with observation and experiment. His philosophy is exemplified in one of his letters to Jenner 'but why think, why not trie the Expt?' Like Jenner, Hunter was a naturalist. He was always probing the ways of animals and birds, in addition to his work in medicine. His later correspondence is full of such matters. The two men became great friends and Jenner met other notable scientists during his time in London. One of these was Joseph Banks, who was later knighted and elected as President of the Royal Society. Banks had accompanied Captain Cook on his first voyage to Australia. Hunter recommended Jenner to Banks as the ideal person to organise and classify the many specimens brought back from the expedition. Jenner declined Banks's invitation for him to join Cook's second voyage, and also the offer of a partnership in London with Hunter, preferring to return in 1773 to follow a career as a general practitioner at Berkeley. Lack of a formal qualification was not a barrier to him setting up this facility in a remote rural village. His list of patients even included Lord Berkeley and his family.

During his studies in London, Jenner had mentioned to Hunter the notion of cowpox as a protector against smallpox, showing him a drawing of a typical cowpox vesicle on the finger of a milkmaid. Jenner's interest must have been revived in 1777 when he met a Mr Fewster who worked

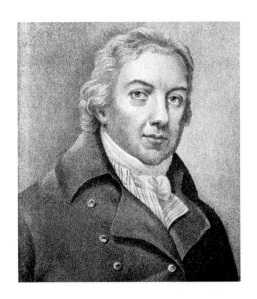

Dr Edward Jenner. From a lithograph portrait.
Wellcome Library, London.

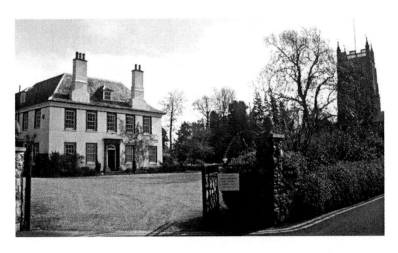

The Chantry – Dr Edward Jenner's home – this now houses The Jenner Museum.

in Thornbury, some three miles south of Berkeley. Fewster had read a paper to the Royal Society in 1765 on 'Cowpox and its ability to prevent Smallpox'. The subject was often discussed between Jenner and his group of medical friends when they met regularly for drinks at the Ship Inn near Alveston. In March 1778 Edward Jenner wedded Catherine Kingscote, the niece of the Countess of Suffolk. They settled into The Chantry, an imposing residence which had been built next to the church in Berkeley. During twenty-seven years of happy married life the couple were blessed with three children. A smallpox epidemic swept through the locality in the year of the wedding, and this may have encouraged Jenner to start making notes about the rumours of cowpox. Ten years later he published a paper on the cuckoo, describing how the cuckoo chick pushed the eggs of its foster parents from the nest to become the sole recipient of their care. He was elected a Fellow of the Royal Society for this discovery. The degree of Doctor of Medicine was purchased for Jenner on the 7th July 1792 with the support of two friends, Caleb Parry and John Hickes. By now the gatherings at the Ship Inn had evolved into a medical society for those in Bath and the surrounding area. Many topics were discussed. Then, as now, such societies formed a valuable resource for continuing professional development, but Jenner mourned the loss of his greatest inspiration when John Hunter died in 1793.

As Christmas approached in 1794 Jenner became ill with 'typhus', although this was more likely to have been typhoid fever. However, this particular cloud was to have a silver lining. After a slow recovery, Jenner took a house in Cheltenham during the summer of 1795 to further his recuperation. Cheltenham was a spa town, where people came to take or bathe in the curative waters, and the provincial gathering-place had become a very fashionable holiday resort. George III had established the *beau monde* when he visited in 1788, so the town's 'season' became a magnet for the gentry from that time onwards. The book by Paul Saunders chronicles this part of Jenner's life and illustrates the huge sea change in the doctor's social intercourse. Cheltenham brought him encounters with the powerful influence of those who were endowed with great wealth and position. Jenner took full advantage of the situation, making many useful friendships. Equally important was the opportunity for him to discourse with intellectuals who were drawn to the town from a wide geographical area. Jenner's many conversations with his peers at this time could have brought him more anecdotes of the cowpox rumours and may well have given him the confidence to proceed. Jenner and his family returned to Berkeley in the autumn of 1795, but he retained his connections with Cheltenham society.

Now came the event that was to bring Jenner fame and secure his place in history. Twenty-eight years after he had been given the notion about cowpox, and twenty-two years after Benjamin Jesty's experiment, Edward Jenner performed his first vaccination. On the 14th May 1796 he took cowpox material from a lesion on the hand of the dairymaid, Sarah Nelmes, and used a lancet to introduce this into the arm of an eight-year-old boy named James Phipps. Sarah had been milking a cow known as Blossom, and had contracted the cowpox. Phipps's only reaction to the vaccination was a slight fever. Reddish pustules, each with a bluish sunken centre, appeared at the site of the incisions. Jenner waited until the 1st July, then deliberately infected the boy by inoculating him with smallpox. Phipps was unaffected and remained well, protected by the cowpox. Jenner wrote to his friend Edward Gardner soon after to tell him the results. The following year, Jenner showed his first version of a paper describing the experiment to two officers of the Royal Society. Everard Home FRS and Sir Joseph Banks, now the Society's President, were both known to Jenner through his time with Hunter. This was not a formal submission. They did read the manuscript but it was rejected for lack of proven investigation. Only one vaccination had been performed. The rest of the text was concerned with circumstantial evidence – his observations on the protective effects of naturally acquired cowpox. Jenner was advised that his reputation might suffer. An extract from a letter of the 22nd April 1797 written by Home states:

'the instances are much too few to admit of conclusions being drawn from them – if 20 or 30 children were inoculated for the Cow Pox and afterwards for the Smallpox without taking it, I might be led to change my opinion, at present however I want faith'.

Two years passed before Jenner attempted further experiments. These marked a radical departure from his single experiment with Phipps. He took cowpox lymph directly from a cow and vaccinated a human, exactly as Jesty had done before him. He then performed a series of transfers of lymph from the skin lesions as they developed, passaging the cowpox virus sequentially from human to human. The diagram below shows Jenner's series of vaccinations performed in March 1798:

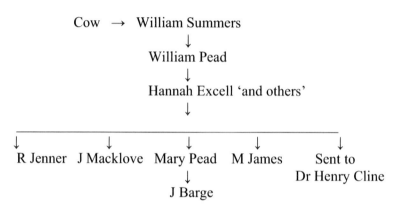

This was a far more methodical approach and is a measure of the confidence he must have had in proving the theory. After a short time, William Pead and J Barge were duly inoculated with smallpox. Like Phipps, these children remained well and did not show a reaction. Jenner had demonstrated that protection could still be achieved after the original cowpox material had been passed through several human to human transfers. He must have realised at this early stage that he had found the mechanism for treating large numbers of people.

This time, Jenner decided to publish without taking any chances of refusal. He paid for the paper to be printed by Sampson Low, at Berwick Street in London. Its title was '*An Inquiry into The Causes and Effects of the Variolae Vaccinae, a disease discovered in some of the Western Counties of England particularly Gloucestershire and known by the name of The Cowpox*'. Within the text, he actually uses the word 'virus', though his meaning – in ignorance of microbes - was 'a poison'.

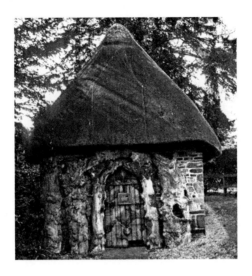

The 'Temple of Vaccinia', a hut built for Jenner in The Chantry garden by the Rev Ferryman to convey a romantic 'pastoral' image of the vaccinator.

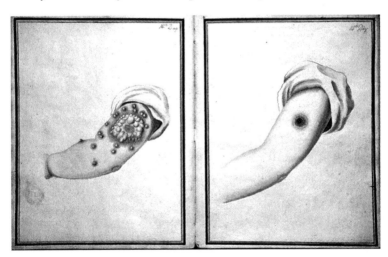

Lesions of <u>inoculation with smallpox</u>, and <u>vaccination with cowpox</u>, at 14 days. Watercolour drawings by G. Kirtland, 1802.   Wellcome Library, London.

Jenner's derivation of the term '*Variolae Vaccinae*' was the Latin for 'smallpox of the cow'. The paper appeared for sale on the 17th September 1798, priced 7s.6d.

This was the pivotal event in Jenner's life. After an initial lack of interest, evidence began to appear in support of his claims. This was entirely due to Jenner's persistence and the support he solicited from notable figures of the day. The protective effect of natural cowpox infection in humans was confirmed by other doctors. Vaccinations by Drs Woodville and Pearson took place in London when a fresh supply of cowpox lymph became available in 1799. Inoculation with smallpox was still in common usage, so there was ample opportunity to use this to challenge the cowpox vaccinated subjects for evidence of protection. Vaccine lymph was soon distributed throughout England and sent to interested practitioners in some other European countries. Jenner's published work was confirmed in writing by others over the next few decades. He generated a group of enthusiastic supporters, though he also endured vociferous opposition from some of his contemporaries. Within three years the *Inquiry* had been translated into French, German, Italian, Dutch, Spanish and Latin. Arm to arm transfer of vaccine was maintained in Britain until 1898.

The *Inquiry* is shown to have a number of flaws if it is subjected to modern scientific scrutiny. Jenner's concept of true and 'spurious' cowpox was poorly presented, but he did clarify this in a later publication. He was wrong in two of his assumptions. He claimed that vaccination would protect for life, and evidence soon showed that this was untrue. He also believed that cowpox originated from a condition of horses known as 'grease' and that this was transmitted to cows by farm workers. Opposition to vaccination was fuelled by the failed attempts of those doctors who used 'grease', although it was shown that a quite different equine infection, horsepox, could be induced in cattle. There were occasional setbacks, such as the contamination of some early batches of cowpox vaccine with smallpox, but Jenner's ceaseless correspondence and continual encouragement gradually established vaccination throughout Europe, America and beyond. Though England was at war with France, Napoleon consented to a request from Jenner for the release of two British civilians detained at the outbreak of hostilities, saying 'Ah, Jenner, je ne puis rien refuser à Jenner.'

The effectiveness of the new method of protection against smallpox was debated throughout the rest of the nineteenth century. The British Government banned 'The Inoculation' in 1840 and introduced compulsory vaccination in 1853. This led to a voluble and well-organised anti-vaccinationist movement led by John Gibbs. Its ranks included eminent doctors, clergymen and Members of Parliament. Many were prepared to go to prison in defence of their beliefs. Compulsion was ended by the 1898 Act, which provided a 'conscience clause' and this Act was strengthened by another in 1907. This is how the term 'conscientious objector' entered the English language.

Had Jenner kept his vaccination method a secret it is very likely that he would have amassed a personal fortune. Instead, he chose to make his knowledge freely available, and worked hard to encourage others to adopt the technique. Jenner was awarded two substantial sums of money from the Government in recognition for this - £10,000 in 1802 and a further £20,000 in 1807. It is important to emphasise that he was not rewarded for being the first to use the procedure. If his petition had rested solely on having been the first to vaccinate with cowpox, it could not have been upheld. When the motion for Jenner's second award was discussed in the House of Commons on the 29th July 1807, Mr Shaw Lefevre countered by saying that Jesty had 'discovered the use of cowpox long before Jenner, and if the House was resolved to be liberal, the reward should be shared with Jesty, or Jesty's family'. His amendment was not adopted. Jenner received honours from many countries of the world and became the most decorated man of his generation. He was introduced to those in the highest strata of society, including some of the crowned heads of Europe, but he was never given a knighthood. His wife's long battle with illness eventually took its toll. Mrs Catherine Jenner died in September 1815. Her husband was to survive her for another eight years. He died on 26th January 1823 after being copiously bled following 'a fit of apoplexy' (a stroke). James Phipps was among the mourners at his funeral on the 3rd February. Jenner lies next to Catherine, beside the altar in The Minster Church of St Mary the Virgin in Berkeley, with other deceased members of the family. Sir Gilbert Blane headed a group who campaigned to have Jenner buried in Westminster Abbey but faceless government moguls decreed that the family would have to bear the cost. No matter. Time was to bring Jenner a much greater legacy - one that he shares with other pioneers and proponents of smallpox vaccination – the complete elimination of an infectious disease from the surface of our planet.

But why 'enigmatic' in the title of this chapter? I used this adjective because the character of Edward Jenner has always been a matter of controversy. Was he a humble country doctor who founded the new miracle of vaccination single-handedly, or did his much-lauded celebrity eclipse the personal contributions of others into unjust shadow? Chroniclers of Jenner, past and present, have expressed marked differences of opinion over this issue. Baron and Fisher paint glowing, adulatory portraits of a simple country doctor who rose to greatness. Crookshank is more pragmatic and explores Jenner's work rather critically. This is echoed by Horton who described him as a calculating political opportunist who obtained priority in the discovery of vaccination through his reputation and aristocratic social standing.

We have seen how Jenner preferred to become a general practitioner in the depths of the country, rather than accept a position of higher professional profile in London. The rural backwater of Berkeley was a much less glamorous option. Jenner distanced himself from the fledgling centres of excellence in the metropolis. Instead of a comfortable and lucrative city practice, the scattered population of Berkeley required his frequent riding out in all weathers to see patients, many of whom were very poor. Jenner's decision suggests that life in his home environment meant more to him than prominence among his London peers. In contrast, his status and social standing mattered considerably to him. A study of his biographies reveals that he attached great importance to his family's place in the gentry, believing they were descended from Baronet Kenelem Jenour in the reign of Charles the First. His wife, Catherine, was related directly to the nobility. Jenner's introduction to the social elite at Cheltenham came in the years before he achieved fame. When it became opportune, he did use his contacts in The Establishment to pursue his ambitions. The world should be grateful for this contrivance, for Jenner would not have persuaded others to accept the concept of vaccination without the support of powerful and influential friends. Gilray's caricatures were graphic illustrations of the fear that humans would degenerate into cattle. Jenner used the huge popularity of Romantic poets such as Bloomfield and Coleridge to counter this negativity and so foster vaccination as a pastoral ideal. The title of Robert Bloomfield's poem '*The Vaccine Rose*' was changed at the request of his patron Capel Lofft to '*Good Tidings; Or News from the Farm*'. An extract from this lengthy and melodramatic opus of 1804 pays tribute to the development of vaccination from inoculation:

'Dear must that moment be when first the mind,
Ranging the paths of science unconfin'd,
Strikes a new light; when, obvious to the sense,
Springs the fresh spark of bright intelligence.
So felt the towering soul of Montagu,
Her sex's glory, and her country's too;
Who gave the spotted plague one deadly blow,
And bade its mitigated poison flow
With half its terrors; yet, with loathing still,
We hous'd a visitant with pow'r to kill.
Then when the healthful blood, though often tried,
Foil'd the keen lancet by the Severn side,
Resisting, uncontaminated still,
The purple pest and unremitting skill;
When the plain truth tradition seem'd to know,
By simply pointing to the harmless Cow,
Though wise distrust to reason might appeal;
What, when hope triumph'd, what did Jenner feel!
Where even hope itself could scarcely rise
To scan the vast, inestimable prize?
Perhaps supreme, alone, triumphant stood
The great, the conscious power of doing good,
The power to will, and wishes to embrace
Th' emancipation of the human race;
A joy that must all mortal praise outlive,
A wealth that grateful nations cannot give'.

The consequences of this clever PR initiative saw Jenner's metamorphosis from an unknown country doctor into a much celebrated national hero. John Fosbroke was right when he wrote in 1829 that if Jenner had not gained 'fortune, fame, and high alliance, his merit would have been crushed or faintly supported'. However, vaccination was already saving countless numbers of lives by the time those words were written and the end had certainly justified the means.

What kind of man was Jenner? Did the deprivation and trauma of his early years colour his character in adulthood? In an attempt to throw more light on the reality of Jenner's adult personality, I put a 'case history' of his childhood before a number of professionals with qualifications in psychology and the social sciences. There are obvious problems in applying modern post Freudian thinking to historical figures. We cannot interview Jenner in depth or talk to the people who knew him. Most of us expect to lead a happy, fulfilling and pain free existence today, but men and women recognised the fragility of life in the eighteenth century. Difficulties arise in predicting common responses to emotional and social deprivation that may be associated with a troubled childhood, especially when this took place in a previous era. Nevertheless, the replies to my enquiries did agree on a number of points. There are external factors in Jenner's childhood which may be linked to the theories of Jung and Sullivan. These also relate to Erikson's stages of social development. Jenner's decision to return to his place of birth to set up a general practice reflects a need for a strong sense of belonging. He is likely to have been a single fighter in achieving his personal objectives. This would have brought a strong sense of self-responsibility but a disproportionate need for acceptance and recognition from his peers. Characteristics of his personality could have included defiance, sensitivity to criticism and episodes of insecurity – especially when something of great importance to him was threatened. Examination of the diverse accounts of Jenner that have been written by his contemporaries, and those compiled by more recent historians, show there are valid reasons to suppose he possessed these traits. This has a bearing on the discussion in the following chapter.

What prompted Jenner to act on his return from Cheltenham after all the years of caution and indecision? Did he hear a whisper that his idea of vaccination with cowpox had already been put to the test in 1774 and subsequently proven by a challenge with inoculation in 1789? Was he told that a vaccination 'experiment' had been performed by a mere farmer; someone who had been impetuous, and bold enough, to take an enormous personal risk in his attempt to protect others? This was bravado that Jenner had been unable to muster – until his return from Cheltenham. Jesty paid the price of intolerance and exclusion. This had precluded the first vaccinator from taking his idea forward, and he had no formal means of approaching the scientific community. He was obliged to keep silent until the true potential of the application of cowpox was realised and applauded some thirty years on. By then, the circumstances had made it impossible for the Yetminster farmer to claim any priority.

It is now time to consider if news of Jesty's adventure did provide the long-awaited impetus for Edward Jenner to bring vaccination to the world – an accomplishment that heralded the beginning of the end for smallpox.

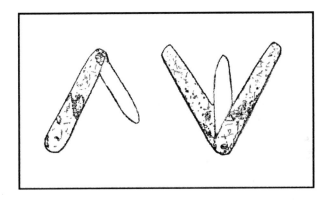

Various devices were once used for performing inoculation or vaccination. The sketch shows steel bladed lancets that hinged open like a penknife from sheaths made of tortoiseshell or ivory. Several would be carried by the practitioner. They were usually contained in a silver case which was covered with shagreen.

Chapter 7

Did Jenner Know?

I have often been asked during lecture presentations if Edward Jenner had been told the story of Benjamin Jesty and was spurred into action on learning about the farmer's vaccinations. Certainly he never admitted this publicly. But did Jenner hear an anecdote about Jesty's use of cowpox and then use this knowledge as a motivation after years of indecision? I have yet to find a surviving document where this suspicion is unequivocally confirmed in writing, but there is cogent evidence which links Jenner with Dorset and suggests that news may well have been relayed by the transmission of rumour and gossip through third parties. I thought it pertinent to discuss these matters in this chapter.

Three improbabilities must be dismissed immediately. Though there were people living in Yetminster in the 1770s with the surname Jenner, there is nothing to suggest they were related or that the doctor in Gloucestershire had any contact with them. Secondly, a Jesty family story that their illustrious ancestor was actually visited by Jenner cannot be validated. Thirdly, there is the appearance of Jenner as an expert witness in the trial of the Dorset murderess, Mary Reed, at Gloucester Assizes in 1796. This is simply an eerie coincidence, for the accused was quite a different person to the Mary Reade who was one of Jesty's milkmaids.

The occasional lapses in the quality of Jenner's 'scientific' reporting must be considered at this point, and these failings are important because we are obliged to rely upon his published work to assess his credibility. Close examination of the '*Inquiry*' shows that Jenner was sometimes extravagant in his claims. The Royal Society's rejection of his first, and subsequently unpublished, manuscript was entirely justified. Jenner was unrealistic in expecting them to accept that the principle of vaccination had been established on the basis of a single experiment. Even the later version of the *Inquiry* that Jenner self-published still carried his assertion that horse-grease was the true origin of cowpox, though he could not produce any conclusive data to support this supposition. He summarised his horse-grease/cowpox theory as follows:

'although I have not been able to prove it from actual experiments conducted immediately under my own eye, yet the evidence I have adduced appears sufficient to establish it'.

With regard to Jenner's somewhat cavalier approach, it is important to emphasise that the 1798 modification of the rejected 1796 *Inquiry* was not reviewed by his peers before being printed and offered for sale. Jenner could also be economical with the truth. His 'Case XVIII' is an account of the transfer of what Jenner thought to be horse-grease derived cowpox from Thomas Virgoe to a boy named James Baker. This entry hides a gross omission. Baker's immunity could not be confirmed because:

'the boy was rendered unfit for inoculation from having felt the effects of a contagious fever in a workhouse soon after this experiment was made'.

What Jenner fails to mention is that Baker was 'rendered unfit' because he had died! Whether he suspected Baker's death was due to causes other than his vaccination is immaterial. Science requires the recording of negative as well as positive findings, but Jenner chose not to include this important fact in his publication. He probably feared it would detract from his successful series of results and provide ammunition for his opponents. This leaves us with an element of doubt with regard to Jenner's scientific reliability and suggests there could be other deliberate omissions in his published work. Jenner failed to pay tribute to Jesty in the *Inquiry* but we cannot assume from this exclusion that he was not influenced or inspired by knowledge of the farmer's experiment at Chetnole.

Jenner had contact with several doctors in Dorset. One of these, John Clinch, had been his friend and schoolmate at Cirencester. Clinch went on to become a fellow pupil of Jenner under John Hunter, and was working in Dorset when Jesty's vaccinations provoked so much gossip amongst the local medical fraternity. He kept in touch with Jenner, trained his nephew George Jenner, and was the first to use vaccination in Canada.

Circumstantial evidence connects Jenner with Richard Pew, a surgeon who had practised in the town of Shaftesbury before moving to Sherborne, near Yetminster. He had learnt about the protective nature of cowpox from talk in France during a visit to Montpellier in the late 1700s.

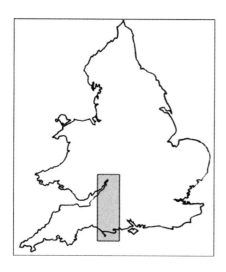

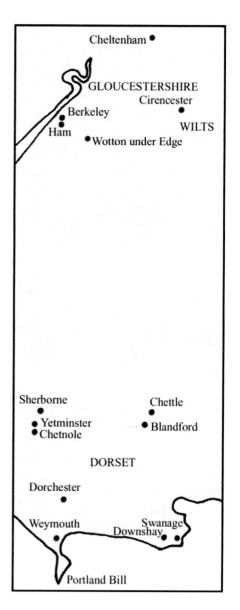

Sketch diagram of an area of South-West England to show the approximate locations of some of the towns and villages mentioned in the text.

Not drawn accurately to scale, but the sketch seen to the right represents a total area of about 100 x 30 miles
(161 x 48 kms)

Cheltenham

GLOUCESTERSHIRE
Cirencester

Berkeley
Ham
Wotton under Edge

WILTS

Sherborne
Yetminster
Chetnole

Chettle
Blandford

DORSET

Dorchester

Weymouth
Swanage
Downshay

Portland Bill

Pew penned "Medical Sketches" in 1785 and a treatise on vaccination twenty years later. He wrote letters to Thomas Creaser about inoculation and cowpox in 1797-8, and is claimed to have communicated directly with Jenner about cowpox, but I found no records of their correspondence during my searches. This is unfortunate because it is very likely that Pew did have a wealth of knowledge about Jesty. However, there are two other Dorset liaisons which may be verified by reference to archived documents. The first concerns Jenner's friendship with William Shrapnell, and the second arises from his connection with William Dolling.

William. F. Shrapnell was a surgeon with the South Gloucester Militia. He was a very close friend and confidant of Edward Jenner. The two men corresponded frequently and had discussed Jenner's interest in cowpox. William's son, Henry, also became a member of Jenner's circle at Berkeley. On the 15th of November 1795 a fleet of military transport ships set sail from St Helens for the West Indies under the command of Admiral Christian. Three days later they were lashed by a violent storm in the treacherous waters off Portland Bill. Several craft were wrecked on the Chesil Beach and there was great loss of life. Among the dead was Jenner's nephew, Captain Stephen Jenner, who had been aboard a ship named the *Catherine*. William Shrapnell was stationed in nearby Weymouth at the time. He gives a vivid account of the shipwreck in a letter to Jenner written on the 26th November, describing his hunt for Stephen whilst the soldiers of his company were burying some 230 bodies. The following year, on the 7th May (only a week before the vaccination of James Phipps) William wrote to Jenner to update him about progress on the erection of a monument to the memory of his nephew – Shrapnell was taking care of the arrangements for this. At the end of this letter is a very intriguing sentence which reads thus:

'I do not believe Dr Graves's knowledge of the Cowpox much more than what Major Tenet communicated to him which were of course your Ideas, but I shall prevent him from making any thing publick untill after your paper appears however, he has just published a Pocket Conspectus of the Pharmacopoeias with the doses, accent, etc a very useful book...'

A close examination of the detail of this sentence raises several interesting points. Shrapnell's direct reference to Graves indicates that his discourse with this doctor (*i.e.* with regard to cowpox) had been discussed previously with Jenner. What is the full substance of the phrase 'much more than what Major Tenet communicated to him which were of course your Ideas?' Surely this cannot mean that Graves's 'knowledge' was simply the folk tales of naturally acquired cowpox protecting people against smallpox? This concept was firmly established amongst country people by 1796 and the notion had already been accepted by several inoculators. The sentence implies that Graves knew something else about cowpox. Shrapnell emphasises that the matters discussed were 'of course your (Jenner's) Ideas'. This strongly suggests the process of deliberately infecting someone with cowpox (*i.e.* vaccination) in order to create the same effect as natural cowpox. Shrapnell must have realised that a publication by Dr Graves would represent a significant and unwelcome challenge to the originality of Jenner's intended paper, so he resorted to a churlish and unprofessional measure. He took the devious precaution of encouraging Graves to keep quiet until Jenner had published. What was it that made this country doctor such a threat?

The diligent Graves was no quack. He was Dr Robert Graves MD FLS (1763 – 1849); a Member of the Royal College of Physicians; a Member of the Royal Medical Society of Edinburgh, and a Member of the Medical Society of London. His signed introduction to his *Pocket Conspectus* dated 25th March 1796 shows he was living in Dorchester at that time, and he is listed later as practising at Bridport in the *Medical Directory* for 1848. His *Conspectus* was published in four editions – 1796,1799,1804 and 1816. He also published a 60 page work entitled '*An experimental inquiry into the constituent principles of the sulphureous water at Nottingham near Weymouth...with observations relative to its application in the cure of diseases*' in 1792. This bibliography suggests that Dr Graves was a committed physician with an interest in disseminating practical information which would help to cure or prevent illnesses. Living in Dorchester, he was at the centre of the county of Dorset. Graves would have had professional contact with local doctors and apothecaries such as Trowbridge, Meech and Paltock. During the run-up to the printing of his *Conspectus* he would have liaised with his publisher, W. Cruttwell (the same as used by Pew), whose offices were at the North Dorset town of Sherborne. This is situated about a mile from where Benjamin Jesty was living at the time; therefore it is not unreasonable to suppose that Graves knew the story of Jesty's vaccinations and that he may have mentioned it in his conversation with Major Tenet. Whether it was due to Shrapnell's persuasion or not, it seems that Graves never published his knowledge about cowpox. I have not found any documents authored by Graves, other than those mentioned above. The 1796 and 1804 editions of his Pocket Conspectus do not contain any reference to cowpox, inoculation or vaccination.

The second Jenner/Jesty link was William Dolling, a very active inoculator who lived in Chettle, in East Dorset. An entry in the *Salisbury and Winchester Journal* during 1770 mentions 'Dolling and Randall inoculating at their newly fitted up house in the Chase between Broadchalke and Woodyates'. Dolling was actually a farmer who had built up an extensive inoculation business and became well known throughout the county for his activities. A later entry in the same journal on the 14th August 1786 notes that 'W. Dolling inoculated at Salisbury'. An undated letter from a blacksmith, F.S.Marriott, to a Mr Newington sixteen years later indicates that this service had been replaced by vaccination:

'Mr Dolling, farmer, lived close to Chettle House, Nr Blandford, near the village of that name and was well known. I might have said that he frequently inoculated the milkmaids but they never took the disease. I was vaccinated about 1802 by an old yeoman farmer, Mr Dolling, who had discovered many years before that milkmaids who caught cowpox never afterwards had smallpox'.

When Jenner gave his first version of the *Inquiry* to Sir Joseph Banks for review in 1797, Banks passed the paper on to Lord Somerville, who was President of the Board of Agriculture - presumably because the subject was associated with cowpox. Somerville read the manuscript and sent it on to a 'Mr Dolland' for comment. This gentleman confirmed that cowpox protected against smallpox but, for reasons I have explained, Banks declined to publish the paper. When the published version of the *Inquiry* finally appeared on the 17th September 1798, Jenner's conclusion contained a reference to 'Dolland' as follows:

'Although I presume it may be unnecessary to produce further testimony in support of my assertion that the cow-pox protects the human constitution from the infection of the smallpox, yet it affords my considerable satisfaction to say that Lord Somerville, the President of the Board of Agriculture, to whom this paper was shewn by Sir Joseph Banks, has found by inquiry that the statements were confirmed by the concurring testimony of Mr. Dolland, a surgeon, who resides in a dairy country remote from this (Jenner's home county of Gloucestershire), in which these observations were made'.

But all is not as it seems. Firstly, it appears that a surgeon named 'Dolland' did not exist in 1797 or 1798. Replies from The Royal College of Surgeons of England, and from the Royal College of Physicians, to my enquiries during July 2004 have confirmed there is no trace of the name Dolland in their respective archives for the eighteenth century, nor were the curators of both Royal Colleges able to find anyone of that name in Wallis's *Eighteenth Century Medics*. Secondly, it is most unlikely that the President of the Board of Agriculture would have been the best person to select a suitable surgeon to review the *Inquiry*, but he would have had an excellent network of contacts to resource someone who knew about cowpox. It is my contention that 'Dolland' was the farmer/inoculator, William Dolling, and that the 'dairy country remote from this' was Dorset.

This opinion is not an idle speculation. Soon after publication of the *Inquiry*, Jenner gave William Dolling a copy as a gift. Dolling acknowledged its receipt in a letter to Jenner dated 28th November 1798. This seemingly innocuous detail is important because William Dolling had been singled out for special thanks by Jenner, and Dolling knew about Benjamin Jesty. Dolling did not keep the news of Jesty's vaccinations to himself. He had communicated the story to a number of people before Jenner self-published his *Inquiry*. Dolling's letters, together with those from the recipients of his news about the Yetminster vaccinator, were produced by George Pearson in support of Jesty before the Committee of the House of Commons in 1805. One of these letters, dated 14th July 1798, is from Dr R Pulteney of Blandford and it implies that he was in general practice in Dorset in 1774. Writing about Jesty summoning a doctor to treat his wife's post-vaccination inflammation he says 'I was not applied to in this case' which indicates that he (Pulteney) would have been in a position to attend if requested. It also suggests he had professional contact with the Jesty family previously. William Dolling tells Pearson in a later communication that Pulteney's 'intelligence came from me'. It follows that Dolling must have known about Jesty long before Jenner vaccinated Phipps in 1796. Dolling certainly believed that cowpox protected against smallpox. He had formed that opinion years ahead of reading the first version of the *Inquiry* at the request of Somerville, and its subsequent rejection by Banks. If there was there any contact between Dolling and Jenner after 1798 no written evidence remains, but it may be more than a coincidence that Jenner changed his approach in March of that year. He began the series of vaccinations shown in the previous chapter by transferring cowpox directly from a cow to a human – exactly as Jesty had done twenty-two years before. Why did Jenner give credit to 'Dolland' describing him as living 'in a dairy country remote from this' in the final version of the *Inquiry*, when he obviously knew where to send a complimentary copy *i.e.* correctly addressed to William Dolling at Chettle in Dorset? Did Jenner make a slip of his pen, or did he wish to keep any mention of events in Dorset out of the manuscript? Was this a misnomer by accident or by considered intent?

Commenting on Dolling's letter of thanks to Jenner, when it was brought before the Commons Committee, Thomas Creaser protests 'It does not even hint at Jesty's or any other inoculations'. Yet at the very same Committee hearing, Pearson produced two letters from Dolling providing confirmation of Jesty and his deed, dated 9th April 1802 and 15th June 1802 respectively. So the Dorset resident who assisted Jenner sufficiently to be thanked personally by him in print, also felt motivated to provide evidence in writing, on two separate occasions, of Jesty's priority in the use of vaccination. It is reasonable to conclude that Dolling must have considered the medical establishment's exclusion of Jesty from reward to be unjust. Creaser, too, appears to have realised the significance of Dolling's input and seeks to make amends at a later date. He counters his protestation with this telling paragraph which is printed on pages *v – vi* of the Second Edition of his *Observations* (pub 1805):

'I congratulate Dr Pearson on having at length established the fact of Jesty's Vaccine Inoculations…. After the alignment of two different dates *viz.* 1774 and 1786 by Mr Dolling as the period of Mr Jesty's casual imitation of the natural vaccine disease, it is now shewn that Mr Jesty did inoculate from the natural cowpox some parts of his family in 1774. In page 6 of the First Edition of the ensuing Observations, published more than two years since, I have asked why we have not 'the attestation of the accounts of Mr Jesty himself'. I did not deny the fact but objected to the sufficiency of the proof, and now that this is afforded, it becomes more interesting to consider how far Dr Jenner's title is thereby affected'.

The correspondence used as evidence in the Commons shows that accounts of Jesty's vaccinations had been broadcast from Honiton in East Devon across the south to Blandford in East Dorset. Knowledge of Jesty was widespread for many years before the Rev Bell championed his cause - quite independently of Pearson. Mr Banks, the Member of Parliament for Corfe Castle, wrote to Bell on 16th October 1804:

'A fact, relating to a farmer in Dorsetshire, which I take to be the same that is mentioned in the enclosed papers (Bell's statement), was given in evidence before the Committee of the House of Commons, to whom Dr Jenner's petition was referred, and, if am not mistaken, was printed in their report. There was, I am sure, abundant proof of the disorder (cowpox) being known, and of its preventive powers, long before Dr Jenner's name was heard'.

My various researches have led me to believe it is very unlikely that Jenner was in ignorance of Jesty. A large number of medical and quasi-medical practitioners knew the story, and it is logical to suppose these included Jenner's associates in Dorset. There were many opportunities for Jenner to have heard an entertaining anecdote about a Dorset farmer using cowpox to vaccinate. He loved conversation and attended many social gatherings in Cheltenham. There was also the dialogue with his contemporaries at the Ship Inn and meetings with his fellow Masons. Something must have led Jenner to act after all the years of reluctance. What influenced him to change his approach between 1796 and 1798, when he began the series of vaccinations with a transfer of cowpox direct from the cow – as Jesty had done before him? Did he attempt, unsuccessfully, to appear in print so soon after just one vaccination in 1796 because he feared that Graves might publish what he knew? Unfortunately, much of Jenner's correspondence did not survive after his death and some loose ends may have to remain untied. Unless other documents come to light and provide confirmation, the conclusion expressed at the top of this page must remain as a proposition, but I have been careful to base this on sound reasoning from the historical evidence that is available at the present time.

Sir Isaac Newton said 'if I have seen further it is by standing on the shoulders of giants.' The true scientist always pays tribute to the work of others by quoting references, but one of Jenner's shortcomings was that he never cited his sources and influences. It is unlikely that he would have given Jesty any credit, even if he had recognised merit in the farmer's enterprise. The impenetrable barriers separating the social classes at that time would have made this impossible and endangered Jenner's professional reputation. There is further evidence for this. Jenner exposed his prejudices in a sevenfold classification of the human intellect in an essay published by 'The Artist' in 1807. He had it reprinted in 1820. Categories ranged from 'The Idiot, The Dolt, Mediocrity' (most of mankind) through to 'Mental Perfection, Eccentricity, Insanity and The Maniac'. Placing Jesty any higher than 'Mediocrity' in this scheme would have been unthinkable for Jenner. He would have been astonished at any hint of a suggestion that Jesty had been intelligent enough to deduce that the deliberate application of cowpox to a human would protect against smallpox, or that he could have devised the means to achieve this. Paying any tribute to Jesty would have greatly undermined Jenner's status, and he obviously took great exception to a mere farmer being fêted in London by George Pearson.

If Jenner had been told about Jesty, he was never going to admit it publicly. Conversely, if Jenner did not know, it is very odd, because many of his West Country contemporaries certainly did. None of this alters the fact that Jenner worked hard to get vaccination accepted by the medical establishment of the day, and in doing so, staked his claim to immortality. The world associates the origins of induced immunity with the name of Edward Jenner because his friends and supporters made sure that the 'discovery' became recognised solely as his achievement. This misinformation still has its adherents, but if we put the received wisdom of our history books aside for a moment and assume that this version of events is not strictly accurate, we are left with some questions to answer.

Where and when was vaccination really 'discovered' and by whom?

L'ORIGINE DE LA VACCINE

This etching with watercolour, published by Depeuille in Paris c1800 is reproduced on the front cover. A physician inspects a cowpox lesion on a milkmaid's hand, while a farmer hands a lancet to another physician. Could the portly farmer be a caricature of Jesty? His act of passing the open lancet to a rather surprised doctor would seem to imply an invitation to undertake a new procedure. The doctor's body language suggests reluctance.

The inclusion of the sinking ship (far left) is assumed to be a satirical joke, but given Shrapnell's interaction with Graves and Jenner at the time of the Portland shipwreck disaster, it represents a curiously appropriate - if unintentional - coincidence.

Chapter 8

So - Who Discovered Vaccination?

In 1998 I read an excellent article that had been written by Dr Cary Gross and Dr Kent Sepkowitz who were working in the Memorial Sloan Kettering Cancer Centre in New York. Their paper was entitled 'The Myth of the Medical Breakthrough'. It was published in the *International Journal of Infectious Diseases*. The authors drew attention to the media handling of advances in science and medicine and the consequent false concept of a 'breakthrough' which is then misleadingly attributed to a single researcher. Their paper explained how this often leads to a profound misunderstanding of the mechanisms of scientific research, inappropriate bias in the recognition of achievement, and a misguided direction of research funding. News of a 'breakthrough' can encourage the public to entertain unrealistic expectations. When these fail to materialise, people are left with a loss of confidence in the authorities. Similar assumptions contribute to distortions in the chronicles of history. Gross and Sepkowitz quoted Sir Francis Darwin (see the Introduction of this book) as an explanation of how the erroneous 'standard accounts' catalogued by Wainwright are created. They used Edward Jenner and the discovery of vaccination as their example of this phenonmenon.

How should we perceive the approach to scientific research and development? The fictional concept of the lone scientist is an unfortunate cliché perpetuated by television and film directors. A more appropriate image would be represented by people running in a never-ending relay with the Olympic torch. Each plays their part, then hands the torch on to others. The relay is comprised of individuals, but each runner is an analogy for a team of scientists. The torch symbolises the ideas and additions to knowledge that have been generated by each team in turn. The teams share their findings by publication, and pay full tribute to those whose previous efforts provided ideas for their investigations. Very few participants become household names. Most of those working in science remain unknown. Their work might result in small, but worthwhile, additions to knowledge in their chosen subject. Often they explore lengthy avenues of research that may lead nowhere. It is a competitive world where healthy rivalry occasionally precipitates professional jealousies, but scientific excellence usually results from a global endeavour which thrives on co-operation and communication. To be fair to the media, it can be very difficult to explain the complexities of research in the physical and medical sciences in everyday language. Editors work to attract the attention of their readers. News of a 'breakthrough' makes sensational headlines but often conveys a misrepresentation of the real situation.

Readers who have journeyed through the previous chapters of this book may now be open to persuasion that the 'discovery' of vaccination was not a medical breakthrough which occurred as a single event in history. For centuries the only means of stimulating immunity artificially were the various methods of the application of live smallpox virus to a human recipient. We have seen that true vaccination began with the use of cowpox. Many medical historians now accept that Benjamin Jesty was the first person known to vaccinate, but Edward Jenner rose to greatness by refining vaccination and bringing it into common usage. Comparing the simplicity of Jesty's rural logic, and Jenner's 'scientific' method, reveals a meeting of minds. These two men came from very different social backgrounds, and although a lack of educational prowess represented an insurmountable barrier to those born of lower status in the class structures of the eighteenth century, there is much common thinking in their approach to solving the problem of smallpox. Both Jesty and Jenner had derived the cowpox notion from dairymaids, consolidated the theory by observation, and used this information to devise an effective clinical procedure. Jenner had the benefit of discussion with his peers, whilst any debate about Jesty's intentions was wisely confined to the members of his own household. Their practical applications differed considerably. Jesty was so convinced 'from his great strength of mind' that he was prepared to perform true vaccination (*i.e.* by definition - from the cow) on those he held most dear. After years of indecision, Jenner used an alternative method involving person to person transfer of cowpox, proving this technique on the children of other parents before immunising his own son.

Both men were unable to explain how cowpox protected against smallpox, and each of them was held to ridicule by the public. Jenner's publications, extensive correspondence and influential support gradually encouraged widespread adoption of vaccination in the face of vociferous opposition. Despite fuelling confusion over the question of lifelong protection and the derivation of cowpox from 'grease', his recognition of 'true' and 'spurious' cowpox was all-important in selecting effective vaccine material. Jesty was unable to publish details of his own venture because he lacked scientific training, relevant professional credentials, and membership of the appropriate social class. His only motivation was the well-being of his family, whereas Jenner – like Haygarth and Woodville - foresaw the potential to eradicate a pestilence for all mankind, and he was prepared to go to considerable lengths to inaugurate this grand design.

Jenner brought the practice of vaccination to the world and made his knowledge freely available. He did not claim to be the first to perform the technique, though it is usually assumed that he was. Jesty was the earliest to devise and carry out the procedure in the County of Dorset. That this historic event took place in a field is a fitting tribute to the folklore which inspired its conception. Dr E Crookshank expressed his opinion very succinctly on page 264 of his *History and Pathology of Vaccination*:

'Had Jenner made a discovery, and, if so what was it? He had not discovered that cowpox produced immunity from smallpox – it was the discovery of the dairymaids. He had not discovered that cowpox could be intentionally communicated from cow to man, for this had been practised by Jesty and others. He was not the first to employ the test of variolous (smallpox) inoculation after cowpox for this had been performed upon Mrs Jesty, and as for the test of exposure to infection, this had been carried out repeatedly'.

Jesty's confident approach to his experiment is difficult for us to comprehend in modern times and his good intentions cannot be subjected fairly to the medical ethics of a generation living 230 years later. We should celebrate Jesty because vaccination has its roots in country folklore rather than in the halls of academia. The Yetminster farmer represents the inherent homespun genius of the common man, a phenomenon often belittled or repressed. In our own increasingly virtual world, where personal flair is frequently dismissed in favour of the inflated wisdom of perceived 'experts', the magnitude of Jesty's initiative and fortitude is something to be applauded even now. Benjamin Jesty should command our admiration and respect. He is worthy of a greater place in the chronicles of history.

I should now like to propose an answer to the question which forms the title of this chapter. My argument will be based upon a foundation of factual information presented in earlier chapters, but the personal opinion expressed at the top of page 99 is excluded. I would like to place matters into context by answering a number of other questions first. I hope the reader may also find this exercise useful for it provides a summary of the detailed content of this book.

1. *Who was the first to describe what we now call immunity?*
The Athenian general, Thucydides, in 630 BC. He noted that those who survived the plague rarely suffered from it again.

2. *Who first stimulated immunity by deliberately infecting someone with a microbial disease?*
Unknown, but a method was recorded as being used in the southern province of Szechuan in China during the Sung Dynasty, from 968 to 1280 AD. The Chinese had developed the method of insufflation – blowing ground smallpox material into the nasal passages of the recipient through a length of bamboo. This form of variolation (the application of live smallpox virus to stimulate an immune response) is believed to have been in use in China as early as 10 BC.

3. *Who first reported the Turkish version of variolation?*
Emanuel Timoni in 1713 and Giacomo Pylarini in 1715. Their information was noted by the British Royal Society but not thought significant.

4. Who was the first to use the Turkish procedure – The Inoculation - in the West?
The first Briton was Dr Charles Maitland in 1718 at the instigation of Lady Mary Wortley Montagu during her stay in Constantinople. He was also the first to inoculate in Britain in 1721. Inoculation was introduced into America in 1721 by the Rev Cotton Mather and Dr Zabdiel Boylston, independently of Maitland and Montagu.

5. Who first realized that humans who caught cowpox were protected against smallpox?
Those who worked with cattle. By the eighteenth century, the beliefs of dairymaids and farmers had become part of the folklore of country people. The dairymaids' contention was based upon personal experiences of freedom from infection, and this was clearly evident in their unblemished complexions. Pulteney noted that 'the disease is well known in Hampshire, Dorsetshire, Somersetshire and Devonshire. It is not uncommon in Leicestershire'. Jenner's friend, Fewster, sent a paper to the Medical Society of London as early as 1765 describing his observations that inoculation 'failed' in persons who had been known to have cowpox. Pearson quotes Adams's book on Morbid Poisons published in 1795 - yet another report that predated the *Inquiry*:
'The Cow Pox is a disease well known to the dairy farmers in Gloucestershire – what is extraordinary, as far as facts have hitherto been ascertained, the person who has been infected is rendered insensible to the variolous poison (smallpox)'.

6. Who was the first person known to devise and perform a vaccination?
Benjamin Jesty of Yetminster, in Dorset, England.

7. When and where did the first known vaccination take place?
In 1774, at Chetnole near Yetminster. Jesty vaccinated his wife and two sons with cowpox to protect them against smallpox. Others may have vaccinated in Dorset after Jesty and before Jenner e.g. Robert Fooks, a butcher living near Bridport in 1787. Similar stories were recorded from

other European countries. Jensen - a farmer living in Holstein, and a teacher named Platt who is reported to have vaccinated from a cow in 1791.

8. *Who were the first vaccinated persons to be tested for immunity?*
Robert Jesty and his brother Benjamin Jnr were challenged with live smallpox by inoculation. Jesty Snr told the Rev Andrew Bell that this was done by Dr Trowbridge in 1789. The archives show that the Yetminster Vestry commissioned Robert Paltock of Ryme to inoculate their local villagers on 21st December 1789 'at a rate of 4s a head'. However, Trowbridge had attended Mrs Jesty soon after her vaccination in 1774, and had been one of the first witnesses. No doubt he would have been interested to observe the effect of infecting her sons with smallpox. Whether he too received payment for this novel investigation is not recorded.

9. *Who were the first vaccinated persons to be protected against epidemic smallpox?*
Elizabeth Jesty and her sons, Robert and Benjamin Jnr. From 1774 - 1797, they were frequently exposed to contacts with smallpox arising from continuing epidemics in the North Dorset area. None of them developed symptoms of this infection at any time.

10. *Who was the first to vaccinate with cowpox transferred from person to person?*
Edward Jenner took cowpox lymph from the dairymaid Sarah Nelmes and transferred it to the arm of James Phipps in 1796.

11. *Who first took cowpox from a cow and showed that it could be transferred from person to person in a series of vaccinations?*
Edward Jenner in 1798.

12. *Who first published details of vaccination experiments and made the knowledge readily available?*
Edward Jenner in 1798 when he self published '*The Inquiry*' paper.

13. *Who undertook the first large scale 'clinical trial' of vaccination using cowpox?*
William Woodville at the St Pancras Smallpox Hospital in London. Unfortunately, some of his cowpox stock is thought to have become contaminated with smallpox. The results of his study were flawed and the incident was used by the anti-vaccinationists to discredit vaccination. Woodville was also the first to publicise the differences between skin lesions arising from inoculated smallpox, in comparison with those of vaccinated cowpox.

14. *Who invented the first technique of preserving cowpox for vaccination?*
George Pearson. He impregnated threads with cowpox lymph taken from the pustules of vaccinated people, and fixed the threads to sheets of paper with sealing wax or wafers. Later, in 1824, Cheyne added glycerol to vaccine lymph in order to preserve it.

15. *Who campaigned for the acceptance and adoption of vaccination against smallpox?*
Edward Jenner spent a considerable amount of his time persuading the medical fraternity to take up vaccination instead of continuing the hazardous practice of inoculation. He met with great opposition at first, but used his friends in the higher echelons of society and the Romantic Movement to achieve his aims. Though it was mostly through Jenner's efforts that vaccination became established, Woodville influenced its adoption in France. Pearson's vaccine threads helped Jean de Carro to introduce cowpox vaccination in Austria in 1799 and later into the Ottoman Empire. The first vaccination in America was performed by Benjamin Waterhouse in 1800. He asked the President, Thomas Jefferson, to support the use of cowpox vaccine. Jefferson gave his consent and wrote to Jenner thanking him for his work, but the progress of vaccination was interrupted when some American vaccine material was found to be contaminated with smallpox.

16. *After smallpox, who developed the next vaccines?*
Louis Pasteur, working on anthrax and rabies in the 1880s. He suggested they be called 'vaccines' in honour of Jenner.

17. *Taking all this into account – who should be recognized as the discoverer of vaccination?*
The dictionary definition of the word *discoverer* is 'one who makes a discovery, especially of something never before known'. By this interpretation, Benjamin Jesty should be regarded as the originator of vaccination because he was the first to conceive the idea and act upon it as a practical solution to the threat of smallpox infection. However, the situation pertaining to his life and times prevented him from presenting a formal publication of the process to the wider medical community, so vaccination would have remained an achievement confined to his family. Whatever the truth of the circumstances surrounding Edward Jenner's motivation to experiment on Phipps after years of indecision, it is clear that Jenner suddenly felt his action to be well worth the risk. He then developed the method of person-to-person vaccination and published his results, before embarking on a personal crusade to encourage acceptance from his contemporaries. Therefore, to recognise Jesty as the discoverer of vaccination would be to overlook the magnificent contribution of Jenner in making the invention known, exploring its potential, and bringing it to the benefit of mankind.

In attempting to devise a totally impartial answer to the question posed in the title of this chapter, I suggest we should put aside our preconceptions and be clear-sighted in our assessment. Clearly, the prophylactic deployment of an effective vaccine was neither discovered, nor invented, by any one person at a specific time and place. We should take steps to ensure that the genesis of vaccination does not remain another example of the erroneous 'standard accounts' discussed in the Introduction. The sun rose very slowly at vaccination's metaphorical dawn. When new light illuminated the darkness at various times in the distant past, those with open minds saw which direction to take and their thinking was influenced by what had gone before. The concept of vaccination would not have occurred to Jesty or Jenner without them linking their knowledge of existing inoculation techniques with the notion of the protective powers of cowpox given to them by the dairymaids. What happened was not a medical 'breakthrough' which occurred as a singular and momentous event in history, but a gradual development built upon the initiatives explored by individuals over a long period of time – rather like modern scientific research. I do not propose this hypothesis as the view of some eccentric 'independent thinker', nor is it mischief born of a wish to be seen as controversial. It is a natural conclusion, drawn from a prolonged examination of historical facts. Many will find this opinion difficult to accept because our need to identify historic milestones with a figurehead is lodged deep in our psyche. The concept of a 'leader' reaches back to the times when hunter-gatherers first settled into organised communities to farm animals and grow crops. It is much easier for us to condense the achievements of the plural into the singular. The 'discovery' of vaccination was neatly packaged into a romantic story of a lowly country doctor who rose to greatness. It all fitted perfectly – a straightforward 'standard account' that the early Victorians took to their hearts – and one that has remained the accepted version for most people ever since. A picture only a vandal would deface with a new perspective!

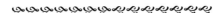

It is appropriate to finish the text with a salute to Jenner, Jesty, Lady Mary, and others from the distant past whose names are mentioned in my manuscript. We should admire and respect the aspirations of all those early pioneers for they reflect the Ascent of Man. Their legacy is our complete freedom from the scourge of one lethal infection, and the means to protect against the ravages of some of the other diseases that surround us. The remaining pages provide brief insights into the death of smallpox, our progress in the battle against polio, and approaches to modern research in the development of new vaccines. This will be my final chapter of a story which will continue far into the future.

Chapter 9

Zero and Beyond

*'And write for ever on the rising mind
Dead is one mortal foe of human kind'*
(Bloomfield – Good Tidings)

It is the 12th October 1977. The scene is Merca, a town near Mogadishu, the capital city of Somalia. The evening twilight fades quickly as night comes in. A man is walking in the grounds of the local hospital. Ali Maalin Maow is one of the hospital cooks and he is about to become known throughout the world. A car pulls up and the driver asks for directions, so Ali says he will act as a guide and gets into the vehicle to assist. Travelling with the driver are three passengers - a mother with two children, a 6-year-old girl and her 18-month-old brother. Both children are suspected of having smallpox. The driver has to get them to the leader of the nearest smallpox surveillance team as quickly as possible.

The World Health Organisation (WHO) campaign for the eradication of smallpox had begun ten years earlier. Using a combination of mass vaccination, surveillance, case detection, and isolation of infected persons, the occurrence of smallpox had been gradually eliminated from the various countries where it was previously endemic. Only Somalia remained as a reservoir, and even there the work of the WHO was almost at an end. Some 2,400 million doses of vaccine had been given during the eradication campaign, which someone has since estimated as incurring less expenditure than the construction of one B52 bomber. The vaccine that was used in the project was not cowpox, but a combination of four strains of vaccinia virus that had been prepared from lymph collected in large-scale harvests of material from the infected flanks of calves or sheep. After treatment with phenol to destroy any contaminating bacteria, the vaccine was freeze-dried and sealed in ampoules. Mass vaccination was made possible by the simple and effective administration of a stable re-constituted vaccine with small, bifurcated needles developed by Wyeth. The origin of vaccinia virus is something of a mystery. The Lister strain has been used in Britain since 1892 but, contrary to previous assumptions, vaccinia virus does not appear to be a mutant of cowpox. Molecular research has shown that the genetics of smallpox, cowpox and vaccinia are surprisingly different. The DNA of vaccinia is not similar to that of cowpox, and unlike cowpox, vaccinia virus does not appear to have an animal reservoir. Baxby has suggested that vaccinia did not emerge as a hybrid virus from vaccine contamination during the latter half of the nineteenth century, but developed naturally after a biological evolution of thousands of years. There was no control over the formulation of early smallpox vaccines. These may have contained cowpox, horsepox, attenuated smallpox, or mixtures of these components. It is more likely that present day vaccinia could be a close relative of horsepox. Unfortunately, horsepox is a disease which no longer exists so we are not able to analyse DNA from the virus. We may never know for certain how vaccinia came into existence but should be eternally grateful that it did.

Ali rode in the car for less than 15 minutes. Sadly, the girl was the last person to die from naturally occurring smallpox but her brother recovered. Ali was hospitalised ten days later with a high fever and headache. He was treated for malaria but developed a rash after a further four days. This was diagnosed as chickenpox and Ali was told to go home. After another five days, the rash was confirmed by tests to be smallpox and he was isolated. Ali had been in contact with 161 people during this time, so the local team vaccinated 54,777 persons in the surrounding area. Luckily, Ali recovered and none of the contacts became ill. Ali Maalin was the final case of naturally occurring smallpox in the world. There has not been any published record of a case since, other than a tragic and fatal episode of laboratory acquired smallpox in Birmingham, UK, in 1978.

Man was the only host for *Variola major* and *Variola minor*, the poxviruses that were associated respectively with severe and benign forms of the disease. WHO declared Smallpox Zero Day on 26th October 1979, after a wait of two years following Ali's infection. Global laboratory stocks of the virus were destroyed over the next few years, except those held at two high containment facilities in the USA and Russia. A decision was taken to retain virus at these centres because new technologies will reveal more about the intricacies of the microbe and its relationship to the human immune mechanisms. So far, animal poxviruses have not risen to fill the vacant gap left by smallpox in microbial ecology. The eradication of smallpox is a unique achievement in human endeavour at the time of writing. This was made possible by vaccination, together with the other measures I have described. Perhaps it is fitting that the infectious disease which gave rise to the development of vaccination was the first to be conquered.

The current plan is to make polio the second microbial infection to be banished to the history books, hopefully within the coming decades. Vaccination will have played a major part in this project too, but the challenge is more difficult than with smallpox. The poliovirus infects when it enters the body in contaminated food or drink. There are problems in making a differential diagnosis of polio in the field. The initial symptoms, temperature and fever etc., are common in many other diseases. Fewer than 1% of cases exhibit paralysis – usually in the legs. The virus is shed intermittently in the faeces for several weeks and can spread through a susceptible population before signs of paralysis are seen. The eradication campaign has concentrated on the interruption of transmission, achieving this through a combination of vaccination and surveillance. Polio vaccine requires cold storage and the ingestion of a minimum of three doses, in contrast to smallpox vaccine, which was fairly heat stable and required only a single application. This makes effective immunisation of large numbers of people a much more difficult task, compounded by the fact that live polio vaccine virus is excreted for a while after administration and has been shown to be capable of reversion to neurovirulence. Despite these biological hurdles, the signs are encouraging. There were some 350,000 cases of polio distributed over 70% of the global map in 1988. These have been reduced to a total of approximately one thousand cases occurring in six countries at the present time. During January 2004 the leaders of those countries signed a declaration to intensify their efforts. The goal of the eradication of polio should be seen as something beautiful to be attained from the application of science, as was the defeat of smallpox. I described my professional background at the beginning of this book. The windows of my place of work, the hospital's virology laboratory, overlooked the polio ward. Each day I could see the patients living out their lives in iron lungs. For many it was a life sentence, brought about by a virus that measures no more than 25 millionths of a millimeter in diameter. Forty years on, that ward no longer exists because polio has ceased to be endemic in the UK. Let us hope that poliomyelitis becomes something that the peoples of the world identify only with the past.

Until we have the option of better alternatives to immunisation in the future, scientists will strive to develop new vaccines to prevent us being plagued with microbes. Considerable financial, experimental and political resources are directed towards this endeavour. The largest project at present is the huge global effort to find a vaccine and better therapeutic compounds to fight the spread of HIV. Research is encouraged and coordinated by the WHO, the United Nations, the International AIDS Vaccine Initiative, the European Commission and governments of many countries. In addition to AIDS, many other categories of vaccine research are conducted under the direction of organisations such as the National Institutes of Health, the Medical Research Council and the Institut Pasteur. There are numerous avenues of vaccine development constantly under exploration in the pharmaceutical industry. Their input is related to need, and the likely return for investment. Although the clinical demand for a new vaccine is assessed in human terms, potential financial profit is an essential factor in calculating the amount of capital to allocate to research. Pharmaceutical companies are not charitable bodies and are answerable to their shareholders. Profits also help to fund future work. There is a considerable amount of scientific investigation connected with vaccine development undertaken in academic institutions throughout the world. Typical studies might include the biology of micro-organisms, their epidemiology, molecular characteristics, component structure or mechanisms of infection. Other research topics could be concerned with the complex aspects of immune system function and their relevance to vaccine formulation. All this work covers a very broad spectrum and requires funding, of course. Many projects are supported by time specified grants obtained by application to organisations such as The Wellcome Trust, The Bill and Melinda Gates Foundation and The Rockefeller Foundation. Grants from countless charities also support academic research, and without these generous resources much would not be possible. The doctors and scientists who work in this field are very conscious of this situation and allocate their budgets carefully.

The public will always be wary of new vaccine products, because they are expected to be willing recipients of 'foreign' material which is visited upon their persons or the persons of their loved ones. Progress of this kind requires complete confidence in medical science and this can be easily undermined. Whatever the potential benefits of this form of healthcare, the reality is that someone may have to stick a needle into us. We endure this gross invasion of our personal privacy in order to combat a greater violation of our bodies by hordes of microscopic invaders. Yet vaccination should be a cause for our celebration. The results speak for themselves. Humanity's well-being has improved immeasurably and the future holds great potential.

Who knows what the coming years will bring? We entered the twenty-first century much as we embraced those that preceded it, with international conflict never far over the horizon. It is depressing to think of the abundance of time and resources that some people allocate to devising hideous processes of killing human beings. In the same decade that the pharmaceutical industry delivered drug therapies to improve the prognosis of those suffering from HIV, someone in the media had a reason to coin the phrase 'weapons grade anthrax'. How unfortunate that the twin spectres of bioterrorism and biological warfare now have to be taken seriously by many governments. The threats are real, and worried authorities look to our defences, but these would be attacks with unforeseen long-term consequences for both victim and aggressor.

This dark shadow must not divert mankind from combining its resources in the war against naturally occurring bacteria and viruses. In that arena we do have reason to feel a little optimistic, but any rejoicing should be brief and attended with vigilance. We cannot afford to rest on our laurels because human complacency is the microbe's best friend.

There is much for us to do - we must succeed to survive.

Bibliography and Sources

Baron, J. *The Life of Edward Jenner MD...with Illustrations from His Doctrines, and selections from His Correspondence.* London: H Colburn, 1827.

Barquet N and Domingo P. 'Smallpox: The triumph over the most terrible of the ministers of death'
in *Ann Int Med*, Vol 127 (1997) pp 635 – 642.

Baxby, D. *Jenner's Smallpox Vaccine: The Riddle of Vaccinia Virus and its Origin.* London: Heinemann Educational, 1981.

Baxby, D. 'The genesis of Edward Jenner's Inquiry of 1798 – a comparison of the two unpublished manuscripts and the published version' in *Medical History*, Vol 29, No.2 (1985) pp 193 – 199.

Baxby, D. *Vaccination – Jenner's Legacy.* Berkeley: The Jenner Educational Trust, 1994.

Baxby, D. 'The Jenner-Woodville controversy'
in *J Med Biog*, Vol 5 (1997), pp 240 – 241.

Baxby, D. 'Edward Jenner's inquiry; a bicentenary analysis'
in *Vaccine*, Vol 17 (1999) pp 301 – 307.

Baxby, D. *Smallpox Vaccine, Ahead of its Time.* Berkeley: The Jenner Museum, 2001.

Baxby, D. 'Smallpox vaccination techniques; from knives and forks to needles and pins'
in *Vaccine*, Vol 20 (2002) pp 2140 – 2149.

Bazin H. *The Eradication of Smallpox.*
San Diego; London: Academic Press, 2000.

Bennett, M and Baxby, D. 'Cowpox'
in *J Med Microbiol*, Vol 45 (1996) pp 157 – 158.

Bloomfield R. *Good Tidings;Or News from the Farm.*
London: James Whiting, 1804.

Busse J. *Mrs Montagu 'Queen of the Blues'.*
London: Gerald Howe, 1928.

Coley, N G. 'George Pearson MD, FRS (1751 – 1828): the greatest
chemist in England?'
in *Notes Rec R Soc Lond*, Vol 57 No.2, (2003) pp 161 – 175.

Collier, L and Oxford,J. *Human Virology.*
Oxford: Oxford University Press, 2000.

Cook G C. 'Smallpox prima-donnas'
in *J Med Biog*, Vol 5 (1996), pp 58 – 59.

Cook, G C. 'William Woodville and vaccination'
in *Nature*, Vol 381 (1996) p18.

Cook, G C. 'The smallpox saga and the origins of vaccination'
in *J Roy Soc Health*, Vol 116 No.4, (1996) pp 253 – 254.

Cooper, A T P. *Dorset Worthies No.12, Benjamin Jesty 1737 – 1816.*
Dorchester: Dorset Natural History & Archaeological Society, 1969.

Crookshank, E M. *History and Pathology of Vaccination.*
London: H K Lewis, 1889.

Davis, H P. 'Smallpox: Jesty and Jenner'
in *Lancet*, Vol 2 (1862), p 461.

Editorial – Dorset Scene. 'Found'
in *Dorset Life*, No. 312 March (2005), p 9.

Edwardes, E J. *A Concise History of Smallpox and Vaccination in Europe.* London: H K Lewis, 1902.

Fenner, F, Henderson, D A, Arita, I, Jezak Z, and Ladnyi, I D.
Smallpox and its eradication.
Geneva: World Health Organization, 1988.

Fisher, R B. *Edward Jenner 1749-1823.*
London: André Deutsch Ltd, 1991.

Fisk, D. *Dr Jenner of Berkeley.* London, William Heinemann, 1959.

Glynn, I and Glynn J. *The Life and Death of Smallpox.*
London: Profile Books, 2004.

Gould, G M. 'Medical discoveries by the non-medical'
in *JAMA,* Vol 40 (1903), p 1477.

Graves, J. *A Pocket Conspectus of the London and Edinburgh pharmacopoeias.* Sherborne, Dorset: W Cruttwell, 1796.

Graves, J. *A Pocket Conspectus of the London and Edinburgh pharmacopoeias.* London: J Murray & S Highley 3rd Ed 1804.

Gross, C P, and Sepkowitz, K A. 'The myth of the medical breakthrough: smallpox, vaccination, and Jenner reconsidered'
in *Int J Infect Dis*, Vol 3 (1998) pp 54 – 60.

Guedalla P. *Supers and Supermen*. London: T Fisher Unwin, 1920.

Hammarsten J F, Tattersall W, and Hammarsten J E. 'Who discovered smallpox vaccination? Edward Jenner or Benjamin Jesty?' in *Trans Am Clin Climatol Assoc*, Vol 90 (1979), pp 44 – 55.

Hardy, T. *The Return of the Native*.
London: Smith, Elder & Co, 1878.

Hardy, W M. *Old Swanage or Purbeck Past and Present*.
Dorchester: Dorset County Chronicle, 1908.

Hart, F D. 'Benjamin Jesty, farmer vaccinator'
in *Br J Clin Pract*, Vol 42 (1988), pp 33 – 34.

Haviland, A. 'The proto-martyr to vaccination'
in *Lancet*, Vol 2 (1862), p 291.

Hayward N. Personal communication. 15th May 2000.

Hayward N and Windridge N. *Badges and Beans*.
Dorchester: The Dorset Press, 1989.

Hayward, N. *Yetminster and Beyond*.
Dorchester: The Dorset Press, 1989.

Hopkins, D R. *Princes and Peasants: Smallpox in History*.
Chicago and London: University of Chicago, 1983.

Horton, G C. 'Jabs'
in *London Rev Books*, Vol 14 (1992), pp 22 – 23.

Horton, G C. 'Myths in medicine'
in *British Medical Journal*, Vol. 310 (1995), p 62.

Huntley, J S. 'Jenner's status' in *J Med Biog*, Vol 5 (1997), p 241.

Jenner E. *An Inquiry into the Causes and Effects of the Variolae Vaccinae, a Disease.....and known by the name of the Cow Pox.* London: Sampson Low, 1798.

Jenner, G C. *The evidence at large, as laid before the committee of the House of Commons, respecting Dr Jenner's discovery of vaccine inoculation, together with the debate: and some observations on the contravening evidence.* London: J Murray, 1805.

Katscher, F. 'Pioneers of vaccination'
in *Nature*, Vol 381 (1996), pp 468 – 469.

Kilpatrick, D C. 'Farmer Jesty and the discovery of vaccination'
in *J Clin Pathol*, Vol 46 (1993) p 287.

Langer, W L. 'Immunization against smallpox before Jenner'
in *Scientific American*, Vol 234 (1976) pp 112 – 117.

Le Fanu, W. *A Bio-bibliography of Edward Jenner, 1749-1823.*
London: Harvey & Blythe, 1951.

Lewer, D and Slade, D. *Swanage Past.*
Chichester: Phillimore and Co, 1994.

Machin, R. *The Houses of Yetminster.*
Bristol: University of Bristol, 1978.

Mantell, G. *The Journal of Gideon Mantell:Surgeon and Geologist.*
Ed. E Cecil Curwen. London: Oxford University Press, 1940.

McCrae, T. 'Benjamin Jesty: a pre-Jennerian vaccinator'
in *Johns Hopkins Hosp Bull*, Vol 11 (1900), pp 42 – 44.

McIntyre, J W R and Houston, C S. 'Smallpox and its control in Canada' in *Can Med Ass J*, Vol 161 (1999), pp 1543 - 1547

Miller, G. *Letters of Edward Jenner*.
Baltimore and London: The Johns Hopkins University Press, 1983.

Montagu, Lady Mary Wortley. *Letters of the Right Honourable Lady Mary Wortley Montagu: written, during her travels in Europe, Asia, and Africa etc.* London: A.Homer; P. Milton, 1764.

Montagu, Lady Mary Wortley. *Works*.
Ed. J Dallaway. London: R Phillips, 1803.

Montagu, Lady Mary Wortley. *Letters and Works*.
Ed. Lord Wharncliffe. London: R Bentley, 1837.

Moore, J. *The History of the Small Pox*.
London: Longman, Hurst, Rees, Orme and Brown, 1815.

Moore, J. *The History and Practice of Vaccination*.
London: J Callow, 1817.

O'Donnell, M. *Medicine's Strangest Cases*.
London: Robson Books, 2002.

Pead, P J. 'Benjamin Jesty: new light in the dawn of vaccination' in *Lancet*, Vol 362 (2003), pp 2104 – 2109.

Pead, P J. 'The first vaccinators 'lost' portrait is found' in *Wellcome History*, Issue 30 (2006), p 7.

Pearson, G. *An Inquiry concerning the history of the cowpox, principally with a view to supersede and extinguish the smallpox*.
London: J. Johnson, 1798.

Pearson G *et al.* 'Report of The Original Vaccine Pock Institution' in *Edin Med Surg J*, Vol 1, No. 4 (1805), pp 513 – 514.

Pew, R. *Observations of an Eruptive Disease Which Has Lately Occurred in the Town of Sherborne, Dorset, after vaccination.* Sherborne, Dorset: J Langdon for Longman, 1809.

Razzell, P. *The Conquest of Smallpox.* Firle, Sussex: Caliban Books, 1977.

Razzell, P. *Edward Jenner's Cowpox Vaccine: the history of a medical myth.* Firle, Sussex: Caliban Books, 1977.

Rutt, R. *A history of hand knitting.* London: Batsford 1987.

Saunders, P. *Edward Jenner, The Cheltenham Years.* Hanover and London: University Press of New England, 1982.

Scott, E L. 'George Pearson: a rival to Edward Jenner' in *Pharmaceutical J*, Vol 259 (1997) pp 1004 – 1005.

Sellar, W C and Yeatman, R J. *1066 and All That.* London: Methuen, 1930.

Silverstein, A M. *A History of Immunology.* San Diego: Academic Press Inc, 1989.

Southey, C C. *The Life of the Rev Andrew Bell.* London: John Murray, 1844.

Steer, F W. 'A relic of an 18th-Century isolation hospital' in *Lancet* Vol 270 (1956) pp 200 – 201.

Wallace, M. *The First Vaccinator.* Wareham and Swanage: Anglebury-Bartlett, 1981.

White, W. *The Story of a Great Delusion*. London: E W Allen, 1885.

Wolfe R M and Sharp L S. 'Anti-vaccinationists past and present' in *Brit Med J* Vol 325 (2002), pp 430 – 432.

Woodville, W. *Report of a Series of Inoculations for the Variolae Vaccinae, or Cow-Pox*. London: Jas Phillips & Son, 1799.

Woodville, W. *Observations on the Cow-pox*.
London: William Phillips, 1800.

Sources

The British Library   Dorchester Reference Library   Swanage Library
The Medical Library - University of Southampton
The Wellcome Library for the History of Medicine   The Witt Library

The National Archives   Dorset History Centre
Gloucester Record Office   Sherborne Castle Archives
West Sussex Record Office

Dorchester Museum   The Jenner Museum   The Needle Museum

The Society of Apothecaries of London
The Royal College of Physicians
The Royal College of Surgeons of England

Ordnance Survey   The Yetminster Local History Society

A much appreciated wealth of correspondence

Academic resources accessed from the Internet

Index

Author Note

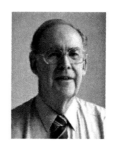

Patrick J Pead has recently retired from a career as a scientist in medicine. He spent over thirty years working on the diagnosis of human microbial diseases at the Public Health Laboratory in St Mary's Hospital, Portsmouth, England. Most of his time was involved in working with viruses. His special interests included electron microscopy and automated systems for microbial serology. He gained a Master of Science degree at the University of Surrey, a Fellowship of the Institute of Biomedical Sciences, and a Membership of the Institute of Biology. These were followed by admission as a member of the Jenner Educational Trust. During 1999 he moved to take part in research at the Department of Molecular Microbiology within the School of Medicine for the University of Southampton. During this period he also worked in Molecular Immunology at the Department of Human Genetics. His personal bibliography includes authorship of some thirty scientific papers, either solely or in partnership with many respected colleagues. He is now enjoying retirement with his wife at their home near Chichester in West Sussex.

Patrick's interest in the origins of vaccination has spanned several decades as outlined in the Introduction. This continuing endeavour has brought him into contact with experts in the field and many individuals with fascinating stories to tell. This book represents the culmination of years of research and investigation. The author is an experienced speaker and has given lectures on this topic to audiences in the UK and abroad. Venues have ranged from medical and scientific conferences to small groups of the general public. The feedback has always been encouraging and inspired the writing of **Vaccination Rediscovered**.

Readers may contact the author at pjpead@yahoo.co.uk